FISH ENDOCRINOLOGY

Fish Endocrinology

A.J. MATTY

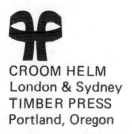

CROOM HELM
London & Sydney
TIMBER PRESS
Portland, Oregon

© 1985 A.J. Matty
Croom Helm Ltd, Provident House, Burrell Row,
Beckenham, Kent BR3 1AT
Croom Helm Australia Pty Ltd, Suite 4, 6th Floor,
64-76 Kippax Street, Surry Hills, NSW 2010, Australia

British Library Cataloguing in Publication Data
Matty, A.J.
    Fish endocrinology.
    1. Fishes — Physiology 2. Endocrinology
    I. Title
    597'.0142   QL639.1
    ISBN 0-7099-1729-5

First published in the USA 1985 by
Timber Press,
9999 S.W. Wilshire,
Portland, OR 97225,
USA

Typeset by Leaper & Gard Ltd, Bristol, England
Printed and bound in Great Britain
by Billing & Sons Limited, Worcester.

CONTENTS

INTRODUCTION

Endocrinology originally developed as a part of medical science and this century has seen a spectacular growth and flowering of this branch of science, just as has been witnessed in other branches of medical science. To continue the metaphor further, as the main medical branch of endocrinology grew, side-branches began to appear concerned with the behaviour of hormones in non-mammalian animals. In 1912 Gudernatsch fed pieces of horse thyroid to young tadpoles and observed them metamorphose precociously into frogs, while in 1922 Kopec postulated that the brain hormone was responsible for moulting in the moth, *Lymantria*. However, it was not until 1928 that a hormone in an invertebrate was shown to cause the contraction of the chromatophores of a shrimp and that this hormone was produced in the eye-stalk of the animals. From this period, and particularly after the discovery of moulting hormones in insects, invertebrate endocrinology developed into a separate and distinct area of endocrinology which has been well reviewed in a text by K.G. Highnam and L. Hill, *Comparative Endocrinology of the Invertebrates* (Edward Arnold, London, 1969).

Vertebrate endocrinology continued to be linked to medical physiology. Swale Vincent wrote a text entitled *Internal Secretion and the Ductless Glands* in 1924 which contained considerable information on the ductless glands of fish although the text was primarily directed to medical physiologists. At that time the comparative anatomy of internally secreting glands attracted much attention, just as several decades previously, comparative anatomy had played a major part in the development and establishment of evolutionary theory. Now it was thought that comparative histology of vertebrate endocrine glands might be able to play a part in medical science. Similarly, in the early part of this century the study of comparative physiology was not neglected, for in 1906 Schafer and Hering demonstrated that extracts made from the pituitary gland of cod produced kidney dilation and diuresis when injected into a dog, just as did extracts made from mammalian posterior pituitary lobes.

Vertebrate endocrinology, however, remained firmly as a 'medical' subject for many years, in fact until the Second World War. This was in spite of the fact that before 1940 noted biologists such as Julian

Huxley had attempted to discuss chemical regulation and the hormone concept in a wider biological context.

It was in 1948 that the first text-book of *General Endocrinology*, written by C.D. Turner, was published to 'present the general and comparative aspects of endocrinology in a manner which would meet the needs of students specialising in the biological sciences'. Research in comparative endocrinology, as it became known, proliferated at this period and the first international symposium was held in 1954 at Liverpool, UK, to be followed by a larger meeting in 1958 held at Cold Spring Harbour, New York. The years 1962-63 were vintage years for the publication of texts of comparative endocrinology with *A Textbook of Comparative Endocrinology* by A. Gorbman and H.A. Bern (Wiley, New York); *Animal Hormones* by Penelope M. Jenkins (Pergamon, Oxford) and *General and Comparative Endocrinology* by E.J.W. Barrington (Oxford University Press, London). Since this period the text *Comparative Vertebrate Endocrinology* by P.J. Bentley (Cambridge University Press, Cambridge) published in 1976 has become perhaps the best known treatment of the subject.

The aims of all these texts were to provide information on, and to establish, a branch of endocrinology which was comparative and general and not necessarily related to medicine. The prime academic objective of comparative endocrinology, according to Bentley, is to reconstruct evolutionary pathways by the study of extant species. Barrington believed that the comparison should be developed on two fronts, the hormonal and taxonomic, and as a result 'we shall hope to extract from the variability that is so characteristic of animal life some statement of general principles which will be reinforced by excursions into evolutionary speculation'. Barrington, quoting William Harvey as an advocate of the comparative approach to medicine, also held the view that 'the comparative treatment of animal function can contribute to the understanding of human physiology and, indeed, is ultimately essential if that understanding is to be reasonably complete'. It was, however, the evolutionary interest of vertebrate endocrinology rather than the medical interest that prevailed with most investigators during the 1950s and 1960s. One of the most interesting evolutionary observations that was made at this time was that of the distribution and chemical structure of neurohypophysial peptides. The chemical structures of these hormones vary slightly but significantly and many differences are apparent between these hormones in fishes and tetrapods. Interestingly, though, the structure of these hormones present in lungfish, which are regarded phylogenetically as being closer to the tetrapod line than other fish, are similar to tetrapods. Also growth hormone and prolactin of lungfish are chemically more like those seen in tetrapods than in other fishes. The concept of homology has provided a fruitful area of research for the comparative endocrinologist.

For many years workers with birds and mammals (other than laboratory mammals) have allied themselves with the needs of agriculture, for example in the study of the hormonal control of lactation in the cow and with the study of the endocrinology of egg laying in poultry. This has meant that comparative vertebrate endocrinology has been mainly 'lower' vertebrate endocrinology with research concentrated on reptiles, amphibia and fishes.

Recently with the world-wide development of scientifically based fish-farming and aquaculture the endocrinology of fishes has taken a new turn. For many years the aim of studying fish hormones was either to support medical science (fish insulin was considered for the treatment of diabetes in the 1920s) or to establish academic and perhaps evolutionary principles. Today, though, many investigators of fish hormones now consider their research to be largely directed towards fish farming and ranching, just as their colleagues working with poultry or cattle see their work in relation to animal husbandry. It is for the student of aquaculture, fish-farming, fisheries and fish biology that this book is mainly directed. There is no attempt to present fish hormones as part of an evolutionary pattern related to the phylogeny of the group. It is necessary, however, for an aquaculturist or a fish-farming research worker to have some knowledge of the form and function of the glands and hormones that control, for example, growth, egg laying and protein deposition in fish.

In this book I do not attempt to define the basic concepts and content of endocrinology; all the texts mentioned above have done this, as have many more. Thus it is assumed that the reader will have a basic knowledge of endocrinology and relevant anatomy, physiology and biochemistry. Finally no attempt has been made to give a complete list of original research references, there being far too many to include in a book of this size. Suggestions though have been given to readers for extending their reading by the listing of more recent research reports, reviews and symposia. It is hoped that those who, for whatever reason, wish to investigate any aspect of fish endocrinology in more depth will find this bibliography a satisfactory point of departure. References will also be found in the legends to many of the text figures giving a further source of information for the reader.

A Note on Nomenclature

Whenever possible both the generic and specific names of fish are used. However, where only the generic name has been given in the original work this name has been used. In a few cases the name of a fish has changed. This particularly refers to the tilapias where taxonomic revision during the past few years has resulted in the same fish being called by different generic names. Today it is accepted that the mouth-breeding tilapias belong to the genus *Oreochromis*. Thus, *Tilapia mossambica* = *Oreochromis mossambica*. However, the generic name used by original investigators has been retained in each case in this text.

Classification should reflect evolutionary relationships, which in turn should help to explain the significance of physiological adaptations of fishes. However, due to limited knowledge of the evolution and biology of taxa higher than at the species level, classification is sometimes arbitrary. Classifications of fishes, taking into account modern knowledge of morphology, physiology and evolution, have been proposed in Greenwood, Miles and Patterson (1973) and Nelson (1976).

ACKNOWLEDGEMENTS

I would like to thank the following publishers and the authors mentioned in the legends for the use of copyright illustrations and tables. Academic Press Inc., Figures 1.4, 1.6, 1.8, 1.9, 1.11, 1.14, 2.3, 2.5, 2.6, 2.7, 2.9, 2.11, 2.15, 2.16, 3.1, 3.2, 3.3, 3.9, 3.11, 3.12, 3.13, 5.5, 5.7, 5.8, 5.11, 6.2, 6.4, 6.5, 6.9, 6.10, 6.11, 8.1, 8.4, 8.5. Tables 1.2, 3.3, 5.1. Academic Press Inc. (London) Ltd., Figures 2.14, 5.19. American Fisheries Society, Figure 2.8. American Zoologist, Table 3.1. Canadian Journal of Fisheries and Aquatic Sciences, Figure 9.2. Canadian Journal of Zoology, Figures 1.15, 2.12, 8.5, 9.6. Elsevier Science Publishers B.V., Figures 4.7, 9.1, 9.3, 9.5, 9.7. Elsevier Biomedical Press B.V., Figure 6.3. Endocrinology Figures, 2.2, 2.13, 2.17, 3.6. Journal of Endocrinology, Figures 3.2, 4.5, 4.8. Alan R. Liss, Inc., Figures 1.5, 1.10, 6.1. Macmillan & Co Ltd. 5.1. Pergamon Press Ltd., Figures 2.1, 2.10, 3.10, 4.6. Raven Press New York, Figure 5.10. Science, Figure 8.3. John Wiley New York, Figure 5.2.

I would also like to thank my wife, Jo, and Tim Hardwick for their help, understanding and patience.

1   THE PITUITARY GLAND

Introduction

The pituitary gland is a neuro-epithelial complex structure which is present and functional in all groups of vertebrates. The part having its origin as nervous tissue is known as the neurohypophysis while that part of epithelial origin is known as the adenohypophysis. However, the possible evolutionary origin of this gland before it is seen in its most simple form in the cyclostomes is a matter for speculation. The fossil record of vertebrates' ancestors to our present day fishes tells us nothing about this gland. It is to the living protochordate groups of animals (*Amphioxus* and the tunicates) that attention must be turned if some plausible explanation is to be attempted of how the pituitary gland evolved. *Amphioxus* has provided biologists with a very valuable example of a chordate in all its simplicity and it is this animal that provides a clue to the origin of the pituitary. If the head region of *Amphioxus* is examined (Figure 1.1) there are two organs which attract attention. These are the infundibular organ and Hatschek's pit. These two structures, the first a neural component and the second an epithelial derivative may be homologous to the neurohypophysis and the adenohypophysis of fishes. Situated in the floor of the anterior end of the nerve cord of *Amphioxus*, the cerebral vesicle, is a group of slender cells known as the infundibular organ which contain certain granules. These granules stain with a dye which also stains the granules contained in neurosecretory cells, such as those found in hypothalamus and neurohypophysis of vertebrates. However, as has been pointed out many times similar staining reactions are no evidence for homology of cells. Nevertheless it is tempting to suggest that here may be the origin of the neurohypophysis.

Hatschek's pit of the adult *Amphioxus* is part of the complex of ciliated tract known as the wheel organ, which assists in the filter-feeding of the animal. In the young, pre-metamorphic *Amphioxus* there is a depression in the superficial ectoderm of the under surface of the head in front of the mouth. This is known as the pre-oral pit. For a short time in development this pit connects with the left anterior head cavity of the first coelomic pouch before forming

1

Figure 1.1: Diagrammatic Representation of the Head Region of *Amphioxus* to Show Position of Infundibular Organ and Hatschek's Pit. PS, pigment spot; HP, Hatschek's pit; NC, nerve cord; N, notochord; IO, infundibular organ; WO, wheel organ; V, velum; P, pharynx.

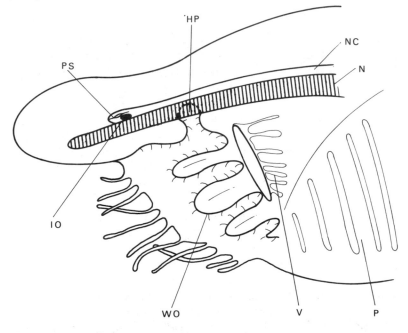

the wheel organ. If one turns now to the development of the pituitary in the elasmobranch *Torpedo*, and looks at the hypophysis it is found that the hypophysis opens into the first pair of coelomic cavities. Thus in the development of Hatschek's pit there is a very similar stage to that in the development of the adenohypophysis of an elasmobranch. It would seem reasonable to homologise Hatschek's pit, part at least, with the adenohypophysis and the pre-oral pit with Rathke's pouch (Figure 1.2).

The tunicates or sea squirts (Urochordates) have also been examined as animals that might possibly contribute to our understanding of the origin of the pituitary. This group possesses a large neural ganglion which lies at the anterior end of the pharynx. Between this ganglion and the pharynx lies an organ called the sub-neural gland which opens via a ciliated funnel into the pharynx. Barrington has speculated that this organ could have

Figure 1.2: The Relations in Transverse Section Between the Pre-oral Pit of *Amphioxus* and the Hypophysis (Rathke's Pouch) of Vertebrates. H, hypophysis; POP, pre-oral pit; LAHC, left anterior head cavity; PMS, premandibular somite; LL, lateral lobe; EM, eye muscle.

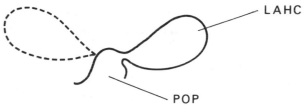

A. *Amphioxus*

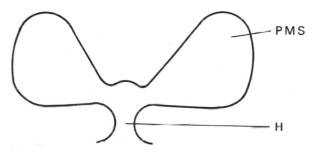

B. An elasmobranch (*Torpedo*)

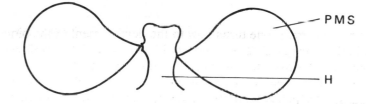

C. Duck

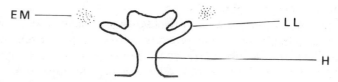

D. Any other amniote

Source: Based on de Beer, G.R. (1926) *The Comparative Anatomy, Histology and Development of the Pituitary Body.* Oliver and Boyd, Edinburgh.

become closed off from the outside world and evolved into an internally secreting gland responding to chemical stimuli from the central nervous system. No experimental investigation, however, in spite of a number of attempts, has demonstrated unequivocally the presence of vertebrate-like hormones in this complex. We have said that the pituitary consists of two parts, the neural component, the neurohypophysis — the down-growth from the floor of the diencephalon, and the ectodermal component — the up-growth or Rathke's pouch, forming the adenohypophysis. However, it must not be forgotten that these two components enclose between them mesoderm which gives rise to the blood vessels of the pituitary. The development, form and function of all these components must now be traced in fishes.

The Pituitary Gland of the Agnatha (Lampreys and Hagfish)

Embryology and Vasculation

The embryology of the cyclostome pituitary has been elucidated by studies of the development of lampreys particularly *Lampetra fluviatilis*, *Lampetra planeri* and *Ichthyomyzon fossar*. The detailed stages in the development of the pituitary of the myxinoids is entirely unknown, larval stages of these animals having not yet been found in sufficient numbers for such a study to be carried out. The development of the lamprey pituitary must serve as a model for all cyclostomes.

The adult lamprey pituitary has a simple structure and for whilst its adenohypophysis is histologically subdivided its neurohypophysial component is even more simple than that of myxinoids. In *Myxine glutinosa* the neurohypophysis projects backwards from the base of the brain as a tube-like structure, whereas in the lampreys the neurohypophysis is distinguished only as a slight thickening of the floor of the third ventricle (Figure 1.3).

The lamprey adenohypophysis arises as a thickening of the ectoderm under the forebrain of the embryo. This thickening or placode evaginates and develops into the neurohypophysial stalk. This is the adenohypophysial analogue which is closely associated with the olfactory placode. As this stalk develops it moves round gradually to the dorsal region of the head while the solid stalk of cells comes in contact with the developing neurohypophysis and differentiates into the three regions of the adenohypophysis (Figure 1.4). The cord of cells forming the stalk remains in this

Figure 1.3: Diagrammatic Representation of Sagittal Section of the
Pituitary of (a) a Lamprey and (b) a Hagfish. A, adenohypophysis;
BV, blood vessels; C, cartilaginous base of skull in which islets of
adenohypophysis cells are embedded; PI, pars intermedia; PPD,
proximal pars distalis; RPD, rostral pars distalis; III, third ventricle.

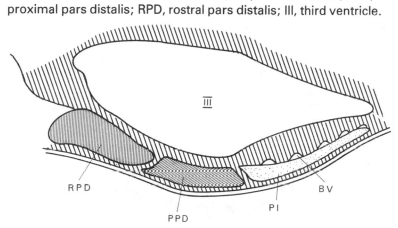

(a) Lamprey

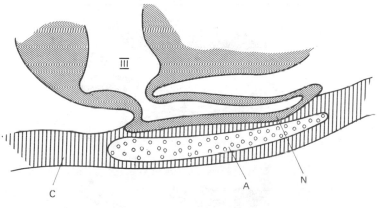

(b) Hagfish

form during the larval ammocoete stage of the lamprey, a stage
which may last for a number of years. On metamorphosis cavities
appear in the stalk. These cavities coalesce to form the neurohypophysial canal which is open to the dorsal surface of the head.

Figure 1.4: Diagram of the Development of the Lamprey Pituitary
Gland with Special Reference to the Association of the
Nasohypophysial Stalk with the Adenohypophysis. a, b, and c.
Ammocoete stages indicating the development of the
adenohypophysial components from the nasohypophysial stalk.
d. Early transforming lamprey indicating connections between the
nasohypophysial stalk and regions of the adenohypophysis. e. The
definitive lamphrey hypophysis after transformation. Ca, cavitation
of stalk shown in (d); Ms, meso-adenohypophysis (= proximal
pars distalis); Mt, meta-adenohypophysis (= pars intermedia);
Nhc, nasohypophysis canal; P, pro-adenohypophysis (= rostral
pars distalis); P + Ms, presumptive pro-and meso-
adenohypophysis; V, IIIrd ventricle.

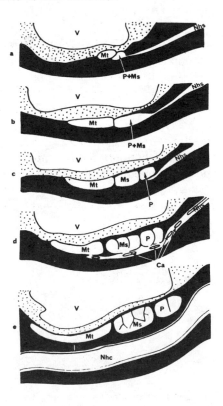

Source: from Larsen, L.O. and Rothwell, B. (1972) Adenohypophysis. in M.W. Hardisty
and I.C. Potter (eds.) *The Biology of Lampreys*, vol. 2. Academic Press, London,
pp. 1-67.

The adenohypophysis of lampreys develops into three regions (Figures 1.3a and 1.4e). Homology of these regions with those of other groups of fishes is far from clear, and at the late larval, premetamorphic stage the connection between the stalk and the pituitary is lost and the stalk becomes separated from the adenohypophysis by a strip of connective tissue. However, at metamorphosis the connection becomes re-established with all three regions. It has been suggested by Larsen and Rothwell that this re-association might provide a significant pool of undifferen-

Figure 1.5: Diagram of Sagittal Section of Brain and Pituitary Gland of an Ammocoete Embryo of the Lamprey, *Petromyzon marinus*, Showing Distribution of Hypothalamic Neurosecretory Cells and Axons. Anterior to the left. 1: ventricle III, 2: subcommissural organ, 3: choroid plexus, 4: habenula, 5: pineal body (parapineal not represented), 6: preoptic nucleus, 7: nasopharyngeal stalk, 8: blood vessel, 9: optic chiasma, 10: rostral zone of pars distalis, 11: preoptic neurosecretory axons ending above the rostral zone, 12: proximal zone of pars distalis, 13: preoptic neurosecretory axons forming the preoptic-hypophysial tract, 14: preoptic neurosecretory axons which enter the neurohypophysis from a lateral direction, 15: pars intermedia, 16: neurohypophysis, 17: infundibular cavity, 18: axons from the posterior hypothalamic neurosecretory nucleus to the neurohypophysis, 19: posterior hypothalamic neurosecretory nucleus, 20: preoptic neurosecretory axons extending into the hind brain.

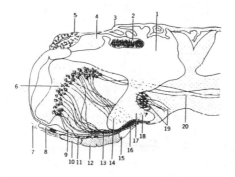

Source: Oztan, N. and Gorbman, A. (1960) The hypophysis and hypothalamo-hypophysial neurosecretory system of larval lampreys and their response to light. *J. Morphol., 103,* 243

tiated tissue from which further adenohypophysial tissues could be differentiated. The pituitary continues to develop during metamorphosis.

As previously mentioned, the blood supply of the lamprey pituitary develops between the neurohypophysis and adenohypophysis forming a plexus with branches penetrating both into the adenohypophysis and into the connective tissue between the three regions. A knowledge of vasculation is important for the understanding of pituitary function. The blood capillaries penetrating the adenohypophysis are surrounded by loose pericapillary connective tissue through which hormones and metabolites must pass. The capillary penetration is complex. The arteries supplying the pituitary are derived from branches of the internal carotid artery and there appear to be two venous drains. Gorbman has shown in lampreys that the vascular system of the neurohypophysis and pars intermedia is separate from that of the pars distalis, and has separate venous drains. He does not regard the region between the pars distalis and the anterior neurohypophysis as being one in which an efficient neurovascular exchange can develop such as one sees in the median eminence of higher vertebrates. Thus there appears to be no hypophysial portal system taking blood and hormonal products from the neurohypophysis to the pars distalis. However, between the pars intermedia of lampreys and the posterior region of the neurohypophysis there does appear to be an extensive capillary network which could allow neurosecretory products of the neurohypophysis to reach the pars intermedia. Electron microscopy studies indicate that in lampreys that there are no neuronal units of any kind crossing between the neurohypophysis and adenohypophysis.

The Cytology of the Adenohypophysis

Before examining the neurosecretory system and neurohypophysis of cyclostomes the cytology will be considered. Whereas nothing is known of the embryology of the myxinoid pituitary its morphology and cytology in the adult is known. As mentioned previously although the neurohypophysis of myxinoids appears to be better developed than that of lampreys the adenohypophysis is less differentiated. For here in the myxinoids this component of the gland is composed solely of follicles and clusters of cells embedded in connective tissue and there is no differentiation between pars distalis and pars intermedia. Indeed it is held that there is no true pars intermedia in hagfish and certainly there is no evidence that can trace embryologically any structure derived from the lateral lobe of Rathke's pouch. It is safer to regard the myxinoid adeno-hypophysis as a single structure; there is no regional cytological differentiation.

Although in myxinoids the connective tissue septum between the adenohypophysis and the neurohypophysis may sometimes be missing, any connection between them, either vascular or neuronal, has not yet been firmly established, although, as will be seen later, a rudimentary median eminence may exist in *Myxine glutinosa*. The conventional light-microscope staining methods for pituitary cytology have been applied to myxinoids and cells which can be identified as chromophobes, basophils and acidophils can be recognised. Two types of basophils, both PAS positive, have been found. Aldehyde-fuchsin staining cells are present and these cells according to Olsson form signet ring cells after gonadectomy. Erythrosinophil cells are also present which show modified structures after certain drug treatment. A characteristic of the myxinoid pituitary as in many other vertebrate pituitaries is that the follicles often contain a large amount of intercellular PAS positive colloid.

There have been many studies of the cytology of the pituitary of lampreys and on changes in the structure and number of cells during their life cycles. Cells corresponding in their response to those seen in the pituitary of higher vertebrates have been found. The pars intermedia of the ammocoete appears to contain many undifferentiated cells and chromophobes showing little activity. The pars distalis progressively develops more basophils during the larval stage. At metamorphosis chromophobe activity is well established in the pars intermedia while basophilial activity occurs in the pars distalis. In the adult various workers have attempted to differentiate cytological differences in the adenohypophysis of lampreys during their early upstream migration and during their period of sexual maturation. The changes are difficult to interpret but vacuolation of basophils occurs during spawning with an increase in number and intensity of staining of carminophils. This implicates these cells as trophic cells concerned with hormone synthesis and secretion at some point during the life history of the lamprey. However, many of these correlations must remain tentative. For example, in the identification of gonadotrophs which in mammals have been shown to be PAS-positive cells of the pars distalis which in a number of species (but not all) form signet ring, or castration cells after gonadectomy. This type of experiment was attempted in lampreys by Larsen but with negative results, although Evennett observed that the PAS-positive cells of the anterior pars distalis become increasingly chromophobic during gonadal maturation and that this change could be prevented by gonadectomy. A further difficulty in identifying the gonadotrophs of lampreys is that none of the cells of the adenohypophysis appear to be ultrastructurally comparable with mammalian gonadotrophs.

The electron microscope reveals one cell type in the pars intermedia packed with an extensive endoplasmic reticulation and with 150 nm granules. There seems little doubt that these are the cells which secrete the melanin-dispersing hormone of the lamprey pituitary.

The Neurohypophysis and Neurosecretion

The simple neurohypophysis or infundibulum of the lamprey consists of a layer of elongated ependymal cells, among which run nerve fibres. The anterior region is very thin and does not store neurosecretion. The ependymal cells of the neurohypophysis consist of a perikaryon and a slender process while between these processes lie the neurosecretion containing axonal ends of the hypothalamic neurons. No blood capillaries are found in the neurohypophysis.

The hypothalamic neuronal fibres originate as in mammals from nuclei in the brain. These nuclei called the preoptic nuclei are homologous with the supraoptic and paraventricular nuclei of mammals. These preoptic nuclei lie anterior to the optic chiasma (Figure 1.5). The cells comprising the nuclei are bipolar, relatively uniform in size and all contain neurosecretion which stains both with Gomori's chrome-haematoxylin phloxin and with aldehyde fuchsin. The dendrites of these preoptic cells sometimes may connect with the ventricle.

The axons of the preoptic nerve cells form a pair of tracts, the hypothalamo-hypophysial tracts which pass along the ventral part of the brain into the neurohypophysis. However, some axons pass into the hind brain as do the axons from the small posterior hypothalamic nucleus present in the ammocoete larvae. Neurosecretion is stored in the neurohypophysis and the production of neurosecretion in the hypothalamic region starts very early in embryonic development. There is no portal system in the pituitary of cyclostomes, there being no capillaries in the neurohypophysis, the blood from which afterwards passes through the adenohypophysis. However, there is a vascular plexus lying between the neurohypophysis and the pars intermedia. It is into this blood sinus that the neuro-hormones must be released although it may be that some hormone release into the cerebrospinal fluid occurs. Thus, although not mor-phologically homologous with the portal system of higher vertebrates the blood sinus between the neuro- and adenohypophysis may in lampreys correspond functionally. Access to the pars distalis, if any, by neurohormones poses a more difficult problem because as we have seen there are no vascular or neural connections. Thus simple dif-fusion through connective tissue seems to be the only pathway — hardly the most efficient method of neurohormonal control of the pars distalis. The neurohypophysis of the myxinoids is a hollow flat-tened sac attached to the brain by a nervous stalk (Figure 1.3). This greater structural differentiation compared to that seen in the lamp-reys has tended to make workers regard the myxinoid pituitary as not so completely primitive and degenerate as it was once thought.

As in the lampreys in myxinoids there are paired preoptic nuclei consisting of ill-defined clusters of cell bodies located above the vestigial optic tract. No dendrites appear to end in the cerebral ventricle but two tracts of axons form, terminating in the neuro-hypophysis. Although neurosecretion is mainly directed into the neurohypophysis some neurosecretion appears to be released at a highly vascular region just anterior to the neurohypophysis. This has given rise to the suggestion that this represents the median eminence of the higher vertebrates. However, vessels passing from such a vascular capillary network to the pars distalis and then breaking up into a capillary network in the adenohypophysis, i.e. a portal system, have not been clearly seen in myxinoids. There is no evidence at all in the myxinoids of the passage of neurohormonal material into or onto the adenohypophysial cells. Neither is there any other evidence of nervous innervation. At least six different types of neurosecretory axons have been identified on the basis of the size, relative distribution and number of granules. This is simi-lar to what has been observed in other vertebrates. However, it is difficult to assume that this means that the axons contain six differ-ent biologically active substances for, as we shall see, there is clear evidence for only one cyclostome neurohypophysial hormone.

The Nature of the Pituitary Principles of Cyclostomes

Hypophysectomy has been carried out both in myxinoids and

lampreys. Lampreys were the first cyclostomes to be hypophysectomised and it was observed that they became very pale and the melanin granules were maximally concentrated. Partial hypophysectomy demonstrated that only removal of the pars nervosa or the pars intermedia caused pallor, while extracts of whole pituitary of adult *Lampetra fluviatilis* caused darkening when injected into normal or hypophysectomised frogs. There is thus no doubt that the pituitary gland of lampreys secretes a melanin-dispersing hormone and it is highly likely that, as in other vertebrates it is produced in the pars intermedia.

Hypophysectomy has also been carried out on the ammocoete larva because it was thought that thyroxine, whose secretion depends on pituitary control, may be involved in lamprey metamorphosis as it is in the amphibian. There is no evidence at all that this is so, but it has been reported that the iodide turnover of the endostyle of the ammocoete larva of *L. fluviatilis* is stimulated after hypophysectomy possibly as a result of impaired ion balance occurring after the operation. The operation of hypophysectomy has, though, shown that the pituitary gland in lampreys influences sexual development and reproduction. Hypophysectomy delays spermatogenesis and ovarian growth and prevents ovulation in *L. fluviatilis*. The appearance of secondary sexual characteristics such as the cloacal swelling is prevented by pituitary removal. The stages of spermatogenesis or the complete inhibition of growth of the ovary are not prevented by hypophysectomy. This situation is reminiscent of the condition in the rat where growth of the oocytes and primordial follicles can continue after hypophysectomy. Partial hypophysectomy points to gonadotropin being produced in the pars distalis but as mentioned previously although PAS-positive cells are present in the adenohypophysis the actual gonadotroph has not been identified. Also mammalian gonadotropic preparations do not appear to influence lamprey gametogenesis, pituitary cytology, or sex characters. Is there then a lamprey gonad stimulating hormone? As a peptide from the lamprey pituitary with biochemical characteristics of a gonadotropin and with biological action upon the gonads of the lamprey has not yet been isolated the question must be left unanswered. Considerable doubt also exists as to the presence of any other hormone in the adenohypophysis of lampreys. Efforts have been made to identify a corticotropin, indeed an extract has been made from the pituitary which when tested in mice had a marked corticotrophic activity, but no hormone has yet been chemically isolated.

Lampreys normally die shortly after spawning but they show marked survival after spawning if hypophysectomised. Also features of degeneration associated with the upstream spawning migration are delayed or prevented. Why this is so is unknown.

The myxinoids present an even greater unknown. Hypophysectomy, and injection of pituitary gland extract have yielded equivocal results in spite of the fact that electron-microscope slides of the adenohypophysial cell structures show cells which are very similar in form to somatotrophs and corticotrophs.

Numerous attempts have been made to isolate neurohypophysial principles from the pituitary of hagfish. In fact, Herring as early as 1913 obtained vasopressor activity from crude extracts. Crude extracts have demonstrated slight natriferic and oxytocic effects and mammalian vasopressin induces a rise in total body water. It is therefore possible that a neurohypophysial hormone similar to that found in lampreys exists in myxinoids.

Herring also established the presence of a weak antidiuretic effect in the cat when treated with *L. fluviatilis* pituitary extracts. Since that time it has been well established that the polypeptide arginine vasotocin is present in the neurohypophysis of lampreys. The evidence, though, is pharmacological, based largely on the work of both Sawyer and Perks, and no chemical studies have been made. It does seem also, at least in the adult, that arginine vasotocin is the only neurohypophysial principle of lampreys and it is possible that this is the 'primitive' neurohypophysial peptide of vertebrates. Neurohypophysial extracts of the brook lamprey, *Lampetra richardsoni*, have been shown to contain only arginine vasotocin (Figure 1.6). The amounts are low compared with most other species. There is a slight indication that some arginine vasotocin is present also in the hind-brain and may reflect the histological observation that some neurosecretory tracts in the lamprey run from the preoptic nucleus into the hind-brain.

In spite of the pharmacological identification of this peptide in both *Petromyzon marinus* and *L. fluviatilis*, in addition to *L. richardsoni*, its biological action in cyclostomes is not clear. Arginine vasotocin injections into lampreys have no effect on water balance or urine production and only a slight effect on sodium loss. In view of the osmoregulatory changes that occur in lampreys it is strongly believed that this hormone does not have any marked effect on salt and water balance. However, pharmaco-

14   *The Pituitary Gland*

logical doses of arginine vasotocin do increase the blood glucose levels.

Hypothalamic Control of the Adenohypophysis

As we shall see, the hypothalamo-hypophysial neurosecretory system throughout all cyclostomes and fish is basically similar with at least some of the neurosecretory axons ending in the pituitary neurohypophysis and their secretory products being released into blood sinuses. In cyclostomes though, with no portal system and little vascularisation of the adenohypophysis in myxinoids and with

Figure 1.6: Paper Chromatography of a Neurohypophysial Extract from Adult *Lampetra richardsoni,* and of Synthetic Peptides. Key: White columns, oxytocic activity (RE – Mg^{2+}); hatched columns, rat antidiuretic activity.

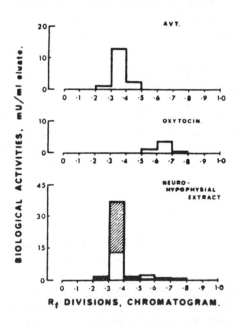

Source: Rurak, D.W. and Perks, A.M. (1976) The neurohypophysial principles of the Western Brook Lamprey, *Lampetra richardsoni:* studies in the adult. *Gen. Comp. Endocrinol., 29,* 301.

no portal system to the pars distalis in lampreys, the neurohypophysial control of adenohypophysial secretion is limited. Nevertheless as we have seen there does appear to be neurohypophysial
control of the pars intermedia in lampreys. Continuous illumination depletes the system of stainable neurosecreting material in
larval *Petromyzon marinus* and there is an increase of material
among larvae kept in the dark. In addition to this possible effect of
neurosecretion upon release of a pars intermedia melanin-
dispersing hormone there is a marked loss of stainable neurosecreting material from the neurohypophysis of larval *Lampetra
planeri* at the time of metamorphosis. This may indicate a further
hormone releasing effect on the cells of the pars intermedia, but
this can only be conjectural.

The cytological demonstration of releasing hormones has been
made recently by using immunoreactive staining techniques. By
this method ir-TRII has been shown to be present in ammocoete
brain although there is little evidence for a thyroid stimulating hormone in cyclostomes. Immunoreactive somatostatin and LHRH
have also been found in the brain of cyclostomes.

**The Pituitary Gland of Chondrichthyes (Elasmobranchs and
Holocephalians)**

Embryology and Morphology

The elasmobranch pituitary is characterised by a ventral lobe, a
structure peculiar to this group of fish, an anterior lobe or pars
distalis, and a neuro-intermedia lobe. In the young embryo
Rathke's pouch is first seen as a hollow invagination which sinks
into the embryo just in front of the oral plate. The hypophysis
develops not as we saw in cyclostomes as a solid ingrowth but from
the onset as a hollow invagination (Figure 1.7). The pouch pushes
towards the notochord to the point of the connection between the
two premandibular somites. The maxillary processes fold underneath Rathke's pouch and fuse so that a hypophysial cavity is
closed off. The cavity lining contains oral epithelium in addition to
Rathke's pouch. This hypophysial cavity becomes apposed to the
forebrain and differentiates into an anterior lobe and a pair of
lateral lobes, these latter probably being formed from the mouth
epithelium while Rathke's pouch gives rise to the anterior lobe. The
saccus vasculosus now develops from the forebrain. The lateral
lobes become deflected ventrally and give rise to the ventral lobes

of the pituitary. The pars intermedia is formed from that portion of the hypophysis which is the original Rathke's pouch invagination while the pars distalis arises from the anterior part of the hypophysis.

If one examines the young embryo of *Torpedo* (*T. ocellata*) the cavity of Rathke's pouch is seen to communicate for a time with the cavities of the premandibular somites via the proboscis pores. It is at the place where the proboscis pores open that the lateral lobes develop. As the pars distalis develops its walls become folded and even in the adult the walls of the hypophysial cavity of the pars distalis are never more than a dozen cells in thickness. As development proceeds the pars distalis and pars intermedia become penetrated by blood vessels. In certain species of elasmobranchs, the more primitive sharks, the hypophysial cavity is retained whereas in others, the skates and rays, it is obliterated and the pars distalis becomes more solid in form. The ventral lobes originating from the lateral lobes has prompted some investigators to suggest that the ventral lobes are homologous with the pars tuberalis of mammals but more recent workers have denied this.

As development proceeds the ventral lobe becomes convoluted and surrounded by cartilage in sharks whilst in the rays the lobe becomes flattened and bilobed. It retains its connection with the pars distalis by a stalk or duct, the length of which may vary according to species.

The adult adenohypophysis is opposed to the neurohypophysis; the infundibulum is a thin neural structure which is largely composed of axonal processes which interdigitate with and ramify into the pars intermedia forming the neuro-intermediate lobe. During development the saccus vasculosus, which forms from the posterior infundibular wall, becomes vascularised and in some species its wall may become convoluted. The function of this structure is uncertain.

The pituitary of the mature elasmobranch is a conspicuous structure lying beneath the forebrain. The anterior lobe of the adenohypophysis is elongated and thin and extends forward as far as the optic chiasma while the neuro-intermediate portion is bilobed and quite large. The saccus vasculosus which lies above the neuro-intermediate lobe is also bilobed. The ventral lobe which is connected to the neuro-intermediate lobe is largely free in the rays but in the sharks it is almost entirely embedded in the cartilage of the skull (Figure 1.8).

The pituitary of elasmobranchs is supplied with arterial blood from two main sources. The internal carotids anastomose in or below the pituitary fossa and branches from this run to the region between the neurohypophysis and the pars distalis (anterior lobe).

Figure 1.7: Diagrammatic Sagittal Sections Through an Elasmobranch (*Squalus*) Embryo Showing Development of Adenohypophysial Rudiment. I, infundibulum; RP, Rathke's pouch; SV, saccus vasculosus recess; TC, transverse canal uniting somites; N, notochord; OC, optic chiasma; AR, adenohypophysial rudiment; ES, epithelial stalk; HC, hypophysial cavity.

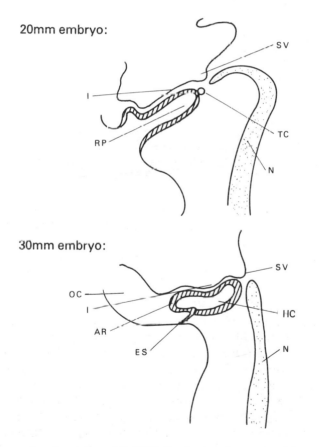

Source: Based on de Beer, G.R. (1926) *The Comparative Anatomy, Histology and Development of the Pituitary Body.* Oliver and Boyd, Edinburgh.

Figure 1.8: Elasmobranch Pituitaries. (a) Diagram of a parasagittal section of dogfish pituitary: 1, Optic chiasma; 2, pre-optic nucleus; 3, preoptic-hypophysial tract; note that it becomes discrete in the caudal region of the hypothalamus; 4, median eminence, containing intrusions of portal blood vessels; 5, pars nervosa, note that many axons ramify onward into the pars intermedia; 6, pars intermedia; 7, adenohypophysis (anterior lobe); 8, ventral lobe of the pituitary, embedded in cartilage; 9, infundibular cavity; and 10, saccus vasculosus. (b) Skate pituitary seen from the ventral surface. VL, ventral lobe; NL, neural lobe; ON, optic nerve; IL, inferior lobe; SV, saccus vasculosus; AL, anterior lobe.

(a)

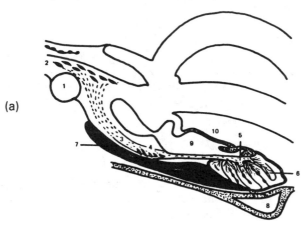

(b)

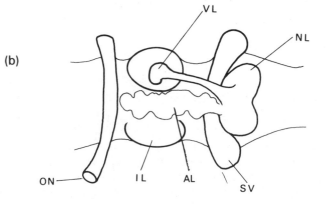

Source: (a) from Perks, A.M. (1969) The neurohypophysis, in W.S. Hoar and D.J. Randall (eds.) *Fish Physiology*, vol. II, Academic Press, New York, pp. 111-205.

Other branches supply the saccus vasculosus and the neuro-inter-mediate lobe. The pituitary is drained of blood by the anterior and posterior infundibular veins and a median hypophysial vein. The vas-cularisation of the elasmobranch pituitary is extremely contorted and complex. A median eminence is present in the flow of the brain just anterior to the adenohypophysis. This blood plexus on the ventral surface of the hypothalamus has vessels running from it to the pars distalis and the neuro-intermediate lobe. A palisade layer of nerve endings, some of which are neuro-secretory, lie in inti-mate contact with this capillary plexus. The fact that the majority of vessels pass to the neuro-intermediate lobe in some species of elasmobranchs is unusual and does not occur in any other fish or vertebrates. The pars distalis is mainly supplied by portal vessels of the median eminence, but the neuro-intermediate lobe in some species is also supplied by lateral efferent veins. Why there should be a portal and a venous system of this kind is unknown.

The ventral lobe has an independent blood supply to the rest of the pituitary and does not appear to be supplied with any portal vessels.

The Cytology of the Elasmobranch Pituitary

As in the pituitary of all cyclostomes and fishes, basophilic, acido-philic, PAS-positive, PAS-negative and chromophobe cells have been identified in elasmobranchs. The functional significance of these cells is not clear in most cases. The pars distalis which can be divided on histological features into a proximal pars distalis and a more anterior rostral pars distalis. This latter region is one com-posed mainly of cells that are acidophilic and which do not stain either with aldehyde fuchsin or alcian blue dyes. These cells have been called T cells or β cells and may secrete ACTH and/or growth hormone. In the proximal pars distalis both PAS-positive and PAS-negative cells occur. The acidophilic PAS-negative cells of this area have also been suggested as a source of ACTH and growth hormone, but with very little evidence. The ventral lobe of the elasmobranch pituitary consists predominantly of two types of PAS-positive cells which can be distinguished on the basis of their granular size. These cells have been tentatively designated as gonadotrophs and thyrotrophs and as we shall see there is some experimental evidence for this supposition. The intermediate lobe is composed of cells all of the same type, often arranged in distinct cords. These cells are acidophils which have a weak PAS-positive staining reaction. Between these cells often occur large osmiophilic globules, of which the identity has been described either as a hormone store or as a product of cellular degeneration. Although the cells of the intermediate lobe cannot be differentiated by light microscopy, electron microscopy has revealed a different structure between the peripheral and central cells of this lobe. Whether both or only one of these cells secrete a melanophore stimulating hormone is not known, but it is certain that cells of the intermediate lobe do produce a melanophore dispersing principle.

The neurohypophysis and neural lobe is composed largely of myelinated and unmyelinated nerve fibres which are neurosecretory. These fibres mostly arise from the pre-optic nucleus. The pre-optic nucleus is found dorsal to the optic chiasma and close to the ependymal lining of the third ventricle. The cells of this nucleus are large, distinct and all of the same size; there is no grouping of the cells into different nuclei. The cells stain with chrome-haematoxylin stain and other neurosecretory stains. These 'neurosecretory' granules of the neuron cell bodies appear in the walls of the peripheral cytoplasmic vacuoles and migrate to the poles of the cells and along the dendrites which connect to the ventricle. The axons of these cells run down in a rather diffuse manner forming the preoptico-hypophysial tract (Figure 1.8). The axons do not contain much neurosecretory material until the median eminence is reached and it is here that neurosecretory material may pass into the capillaries. The axons passing along the thin infundibular wall are of a number of different forms, some of which appear to be non-secretory. The neural lob, closely apposed to the intermediate lobe in some species of elasmobranchs, is well defined and composed of glial elements and neurosecretory fibre endings and can be thought of as a true pars nervosa. In other species the neural elements penetrate very diffusely between the pars intermedia cells so that there is no well-defined pars nervosa. Neurosecretory nerves make direct contact with pars intermedia cells as well as with the blood plexus of this area. Thus, both direct neural and vascular mediated neuro-secretory innervation of the intermedia cells may take place.

Two neuro-secretory fibres have been identified in the neuro-intermedia by electron-microscopy and it has been suggested on this basis that there may be separate control of synthesis and release from the intermedia cells.

The Hormones of the Adenohypophysis

There is, as we have seen, cytological evidence for the presence of a number of elasmobranch adenohypophysial hormones and evidence of their presence by surgical hypophysectomy has been provided. Dodd and his colleagues removed the ventral lobe from the lesser spotted dogfish *Scyliorhinus canicula* and demonstrated that after this operation long-term ovarian regression occurred in females and there was inhibition of spermatogenesis in males. Removal of the anterior or neuro-intermediate lobes has no effect on reproduction. Removal of the anterior plus the neuro-intermediate lobes of the pituitary also delays the disappearance of vitellogenin from the plasma of *S. canicula* but not the rate of vitellogenin formation. It has been suggested that in view of this there might be a pituitary hormone in oviparous elasmobranchs that stimulates the uptake of vitellogenin by growing ovarian follicles. With one exception, removal of the pituitary has not clearly established the presence of other pituitary hormones in sharks and rays. Hypophysectomy does not, for example, cause any change in thyroid histology although, as will be seen, it is probable that TSH is produced in the ventral lobe.

The presence of a melanocyte-stimulating hormone (MSH) has been demonstrated in elasmobranchs largely by the fact that removal of the neuro-intermediate lobe results in blanching of the skin. This experiment was first conducted with *Mustelis canis* but has since been repeated on a number of species. Elasmobranchs show great variation in the time that they take to adapt their skin colouration to light or dark backgrounds and the ray, *Raja clavata*, does indeed show no colour change when transferred from a dark background to a light one. But even in this species, like all others, hypophysectomy results in skin blanching. Further, good evidence for a darkening hormone, a melanocyte-stimulating or a melanophore-dispersing hormone is provided by taking blood from dark animals and injecting this blood into pale skinned, white background, or hypophysectomised fish. The region around the injection darkens and this provides a clear indication of such a hormone in the blood.

The biochemistry and physiology of the elasmobranch pituitary hormones are incompletely known.

ACTH. The role of this hormone has not been clearly established. Hypophysectomy of *Scyliorhinus canicula* appears to have no effect on its adrenocortical tissue even after one year. Also, removal of the pituitary has no significant effect on carbohydrate metabolism. Nevertheless, injections of mammalian ACTH do increase circulating glucose levels, suggesting a corticosteroid response to this hormone. That a pituitary-adrenocortical axis does exist is given some support from the fact that ACTH has been isolated from the dogfish *Squalus acanthias*. It has 15 per cent of the potency of human ACTH in promoting corticosteroidogenesis in isolated rat adrenal cells. The amino acid sequence has been determined (Figure 1.9) and it has been found that the N-terminal tridecapeptide sequence is identical with dogfish α-MSH. When compared with human ACTH it is found that there are eleven differences in amino acids but nine occur in a region of the molecule which is considered not essential for the hormone's steroidogenic activity. A peptide identical with the 18-39 portion of this ACTH molecule has been isolated from the neuro-intermediate lobe of the pituitary where α-MSH is found and so it seems likely that ACTH is also a precursor of α-MSH in elasmobranchs.

MSH. This hormone, or rather hormones, is known to exist as several distinct entities i.e., α-MSH, β-MSH and γ-MSH (Figure 1.9) in elasmobranchs. Dogfish (*Squalus acanthias*) MSH has about 1 per cent of the potency of mammalian α-MSH when tested on frog and dogfish skin. MSH plays an important part in the colour changes that occur in many sharks and rays depending on the shade of the background as previously mentioned. The release of the MSH(s), resulting in the dispersion of melanosomes in the dermal melanophores, appears to be due to the absence of hypothalamic neural inhibiting control.

TSH. Although the amino acid sequence has not been completed there is good evidence for the presence of this molecule in the pituitary of elasmobranchs. The hormone appears to be produced largely in the ventral lobe. If ventral lobe homogenates are incubated with thyroid glands there is an increase in release of thyroxine.

LH and FSH. Our knowledge of pituitary-gonad relationships in elasmobranchs is due largely to the work of Dodd and his colleagues. The ventral lobe of the dogfish, *Scyliorhinus canicula*, was shown some years ago to contain a significant amount of

Figure 1.9: Comparison of Amino Acid Sequences of Dogfish and Salmon MSH with Related Mammalian Peptides.

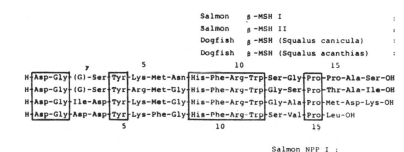

Salmon   ACTH I (1-20)   :
Salmon   ACTH II(1-20)   :
Dogfish   ACTH (1-20)   :
Mammalian ACTH (1-20)   :

```
                          5              10                15              20
H┤Ser-Tyr-Ser-Met-Glu-His-Phe-Arg-Trp-Gly-Lys-Pro├Val┤Gly├K/R-K/R-K/R┤Arg-Pro├
H┤Ser-Tyr-Ser-Met-Glu-His-Phe-Arg-Trp-Gly-Lys-Pro├Ile┤Gly├His-K/R-K/R┤Arg-Pro├
H┤Ser-Tyr-Ser-Met-Glu-His-Phe-Arg-Trp-Gly-Lys-Pro├Met┤Gly├Arg-Lys-Arg┤Arg-Pro├
H┤Ser-Tyr-Ser-Met-Glu-His-Phe-Arg-Trp-Gly-Lys-Pro├Val┤Gly├Lys-Lys-Arg┤Arg-Pro├
```

Salmon β-MSH I   :
Salmon β-MSH II   :
Dogfish β-MSH (Squalus canicula)   :
Dogfish β-MSH (Squalus acanthias)   :

```
         γ         5                    10                  15
H┤Asp-Gly├(G)-Ser┤Tyr├Lys-Met-Asn┤His-Phe-Arg-Trp├Ser-Gly┤Pro├Pro-Ala-Ser-OH
H┤Asp-Gly├(G)-Ser┤Tyr├Arg-Met-Gly┤His-Phe-Arg-Trp├Gly-Ser┤Pro├Thr-Ala-Ile-OH
H┤Asp-Gly├Ile-Asp┤Tyr├Lys-Met-Gly┤His-Phe-Arg-Trp├Gly-Ala┤Pro├Met-Asp-Lys-OH
H┤Asp-Gly├Asp-Asp┤Tyr├Lys-Phe-Gly┤His-Phe-Arg-Trp├Ser-Val┤Pro├Leu-OH
                   5                    10                  15
```

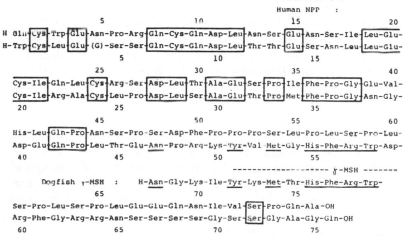

```
                                              Salmon NPP I :
                                              Human NPP    :
                      5              10              15              20
H  Glu┤Cys├Trp┤Glu├Asn-Pro-Arg┤Gln-Cys-Gln-Asp-Leu├Asn-Ser┤Glu├Asn-Ser-Ile┤Leu-Glu-
H-Trp┤Cys├Leu┤Glu├(G)-Ser-Ser┤Gln-Cys-Gln-Asp-Leu├Thr-Thr┤Glu├Ser-Asn-Leu┤Leu-Glu-
                      5              10              15

       25              30              35              40
Cys-Ile┤Gln-Leu┤Cys├Arg-Ser┤Asp-Leu├Thr┤Ala-Glu┤Ser┤Pro├Ile┤Phe-Pro-Gly├Glu-Val-
Cys-Ile┤Arg-Ala┤Cys├Leu-Pro┤Asp-Leu├Ser┤Ala-Glu┤Thr┤Pro├Met┤Phe-Pro-Gly┤Asn-Gly-
 20              25              30              35

       45              50              55              60
His-Leu┤Gln-Pro├Asn-Ser-Pro-Ser-Asp-Phe-Pro-Pro-Pro-Ser-Leu-Pro-Leu-Ser-Pro-Leu-
Asp-Glu┤Gln-Pro├Leu-Thr-Glu-Asn-Pro-Arg-Lys-Tyr-Val Met-Gly-His-Phe-Arg-Trp-Asp-
 40              45              50              55

                               ------------------- γ-MSH ------
          Dogfish γ-MSH  :   H-Asn-Gly-Lys-Ile-Tyr-Lys-Met-Thr-His-Phe-Arg-Trp-
               65              70              75
Ser-Pro-Leu-Ser-Pro-Leu-Glu-Glu-Gln-Asn-Ile-Val┤Ser├Pro-Gln-Ala-OH
Arg-Phe-Gly-Arg-Arg-Asn-Ser-Ser-Ser-Ser-Gly-Ser┤Ser├Gly-Ala-Gly-Gln-OH
 60              65              70              75
```

Source: Kawauchi, H. *et al.* (1984) Chemical and biological characterization of salmon melanocyte stimulating hormones. *Gen. Comp. Endocrinol., 53,* 37.

gonadotrophic activity. Whereas removal of the ventral pituitary lobe causes testes breakdown, injection of mammalian HCG and PMSG fail to mitigate this effect. Thus there is indication of species specificity. When the ventral lobe extracts are highly purified by chromatography two peaks of gonadotropin appear, but both peaks have the same biological activity, that is they are very potent in stimulating steroidogenesis by both avian and turtle testicular cells. The gonadotropin(s) behave somewhat like mammalian FSH when assayed pharmacologically. The hormone prepared from dogfish when injected into hypophysectomised animals of the same species causes a highly significant rise in plasma androgens.

GH. Growth hormone has been isolated from one elasmobranch but its amino acid sequence has not yet been determined. Extracts of elasmobranch pituitary promote growth and are diabetogenic, but are not effective in promoting growth in mammals.

Prolactin. Immunological and electrophoretic studies of the pars distalis of the blue shark *Prionace glauca* have indicated the presence of a prolactin-like molecule. The presence of this molecule has also been indicated in the rostral pars distalis of several other elasmobranchs. Removal of the rostral lobe of the pars distalis in the euryhaline stingray *Daryatis sabina* causes a significant increase in plasma osmolarity, urea and sodium concentrations. Mammalian prolactin reverses these effects. Thus, a sodium saving hormone appears to exist in this elasmobranch's pituitary but other work on *Scyliorhinus* has not been able to demonstrate any salt retaining factor.

Hypothalamic Hormones. Although a number of releasing or inhibiting hypothalamic peptides have been identified in cartilaginous fish their physiological role and pathways of reaching their adenohypophysial effector cells is generally obscure. As has been explained this group of fish have a well-developed median eminence co-extensive with an elongated pars distalis but, in some species at least, there is a well-developed direct innervation of the secreting cells of the pars intermedia. Also, the ventral lobe often appears to be isolated from the rest of the pituitary and have no vascular or nervous relationship with the hypothalamus.

The evidence for a thyroid releasing hormone is indirect, based on the somewhat tenuous evidence which assumes that the release of TSH is mediated at least in part by adenyl cyclase. How (if indeed this factor does exist) it reaches the ventral lobe, except perhaps via peripheral circulation, is unknown.

Somatostatin has, by radioimmunoassay, been identified in the brain of both sharks and rays. Somatostatin, the growth hormone release inhibiting factor, is widely distributed throughout the brain but no direct effect on somatotrophs or GH release has yet been demonstrated.

The Hormones of the Neurohypophysis

Oxytocic, milk ejection, and antidiuretic activities are all pharmacological characteristics of the neuro-intermediate lobe of elasmobranchs. As with cyclostomes these properties were early identified. Rat vasopressor assays sometimes proved difficult to demonstrate, but it is now well established that all these pharmacological properties of the mammalian hormones oxytocin and vasopressin are the result of the presence in elasmobranchs of four neurohypophysial peptides. They are arginine vasotocin (AVT), valitocin (VLT), aspartocin (AST), and glumitocin (GLT) (Table 1.1). Arginine vasotocin appears to be present in all cartilaginous fish but the presence of the others is not found in all species or even in different individuals of the same species. Generally speaking though, arginine vasotocin appears to be present in much lower amounts than the other three hormones although neurohypophysial hormones in all groups of fish are low compared with other vertebrates, when expressed as moles per kilogram of body weight. Also, the detection of neurohypophysial hormones has not been made in the circulation of fish and therefore peripheral physiological effects are quite problematic although in bony fish, as we shall see later, changes in salinity or reproductive state induce changes in pituitary levels of arginine vasotocin.

The injection of arginine vasotocin or neurohypophysial extracts does not affect water balance in elasmobranchs. However, when this peptide was tested in the lip shark, *Hemiscyllium plagiosum* for its effect on arterial blood pressure, a rise was detected both in the ventral and dorsal aortae. It was suggested that this effect was due to peripheral vasoconstriction. The possible function of the other neural peptides found in elasmobranchs is uncertain although they may be involved in the regulation of MSH secretion. This is not though very likely as glumitocin and vasotocin are without either an inhibitory or stimulatory effect on MSH in the frog. It

Table 1:1: Amino Acid Sequences of Neurohypophysial Hormones

Common structure (Variations in positions 3, 4, and 8 indicated by (X))	1 Cys	2 Tyr	3 (X)	4 (X)	5 Asn	6 Cys	7 Pro	8 (X)	9 Gly(NH₂)
Basic peptides			Amino acids in position						
			3		4			8	
Arginine vasopressin (AVP)			Phe		Gln			Arg	
Lysine vasopressin (LVP)			Phe		Gln			Lys	
Arginine vasotocin (AVT)			Ile		Gln			Arg	
Neutral (—oxytocin-like) peptides									
Oxytocin			Ile		Gln			Leu	
Mesotocin			ile		Gln			Ile	
Isotocin (= ichthyotocin)			Ile		Ser			Ile	
Glumitocin (GLT)			Ile		Ser			Gln	
Valitocin (VLT)			Ile		Gln			Val	
Aspartocin (AST)			Ile		Asn			Leu	

Source: Heller, H. (1974) 'Molecular aspects of comparative endocrinology', *Gen. Comp. Endocrinol., 22,* 315.

is more probable that as arginine vasotocin has been shown in a number of vertebrates, including cyclostomes, to bring about hyperglycaemia and an increase in free fatty acids then its glucogenic and lipolytic effects may also be seen in elasmobranchs.

The Holocephalian Pituitary

This group of chondrichthian fish has an hypophysis similar to that of the elasmobranchs. Both the European ratfish *Chimaera monstrosa* and its North American counterpart *Hydrolagus colliei* are characterised by having in the median line of the palate a peculiar aggregate of many follicles buried in a large mass of lymphoid tissue. This part of the pituitary which is called the 'Rachendachhypophyse' is separated in the adult by a layer of cartilage. A cord of epithelial cells does, however, join this structure to the pars distalis in the young animal and so it is likely to be the homologue of the ventral lobe of the elasmobranchs (Figure 1.10). Also the Rachendachhypophyse originates from an evaginated outgrowth of invaginated buccal ectoderm.

As in the elasmobranchs the pituitary can be divided into four components, the rostral pars distalis, proximal pars distalis, neurointermediate lobe, and the Rachendachhypophyse. This latter component of the pituitary is a large compact well-vascularised

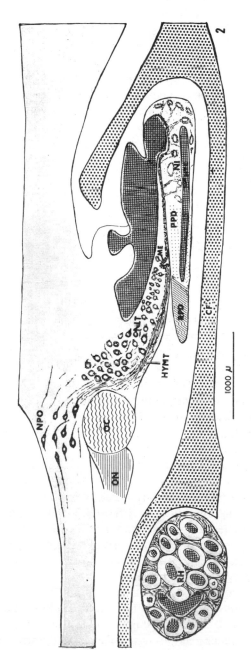

Figure 1.10: Diagrammatic Representation of a Median Sagittal Section Passing through the Brain of an Adult *Hydrolagus*, Showing the Hypothalamo-hypophysial Neurosecretory System. The large follicular Rachendachhypophyse may be noted. CF, cartilaginous floor of skull; HYNT, hypothalamo-hypophysial neural tract; ME, median eminence; NI, neuro-intermediate lobe; PPD, posterior pars distalis; RPD, rostral pars distalis; RH, 'Rachendachhypophyse'; ON, optic nerve; OC, optic chiasma; NPO, nucleus preoptius; NLT, nucleus latero-tuberalis.

Source: Sathyanesan, A.G. (1965) The hypophysis and hypothalamo-hypophysial system in the Chimaeroid fish *Hydrolagus colliei* with a note on their vascularization. *J. Morphol.*, *116*, 413.

organ made up of follicles and cysts. The lumen of the follicles contain PAS-positive material. As in many elasmobranchs the pars distalis is lobulated and is made up of acidophil and chromophobe cells. In the neuro-intermediate lobe AF-positive cells, acidophils, chromophobes and ganglionic cells are present. There is a distinct hypothalamo-hypophysial neurosecretory system, the cells of the nuclear preopticus being located anteriodorsally to the optic chiasma. As in the sharks a few of the neurosecretory axons extend into and beyond the neuro-intermediate lobe, and some even enter the saccus vasculosus. Their function is unknown. There is evidence for a portal system with a median eminence. The Rachendachhypophyse is independently vascularised. Nothing is known of the function or hormone components of the ratfish adenohypophysis but extracts of the pituitary have, by pharmacological assay, indicated the presence of 'oxytocin' and argininevasotocin.

The Pituitary Gland of the Osteichthyes

The major class of living fish are the Osteichthyes, or bony fishes, which have continually increased in importance since their inception in early Palaeozoic times. There are three major groups of bony fishes, the lobe fins or crossopterygians important as the ancestral line leading to tetrapods, the lungfish or dipnoians and the rayfish or actinopterygians.

The Crossopterygii

Although this group appeared in Devonian times, and there are about 55 extinct genera, there is only one living species, the coelocanth *Latimeria chalumnae*. The pituitary of this fish has been described by Lagois and by van Kemenade.

The structure of the gland shows features which are both unique to the species and which are shared with other osteichthians. The most striking feature of the gland is a peculiar elongation of the pars distalis (Figure 1.11). Also the pars distalis, unlike that of other bony fish is represented by two physically separated components with distinct vascularisation. The proximal portion of the pars distalis is again divided into a dorsal lobe and a posterior lobe. The rostral division is peculiar in that it is connected to the rest of the pars distalis only by a tubular hypophysial cavity and consists

Figure 1.11: Diagrammatic Sagittal Sections of Pituitaries of the Coelocanth, *Latimeria*, and of the Primitive Actinopterygian, *Amia*. PL, posterior lobe; DL, dorsal lobe; N, neurohypophysis; IL, intermediate lobe; RL, rostral lobe; C, hypophysial cavity; RPD, rostral pars distalis; PPD, proximal pars distalis (? = rostral lobe of *Latimeria*).

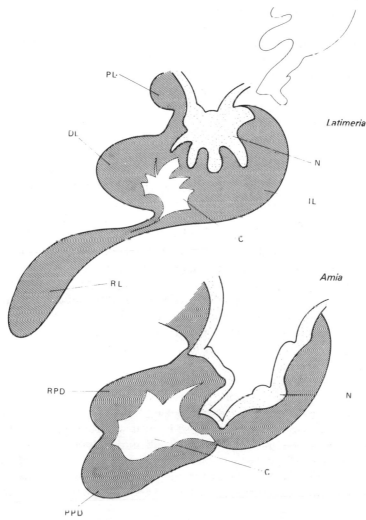

Source: Based on Lagios, M.D. (1975) The pituitary gland of the coelocanth, *Latimeria chalumnae*, Smith. *Gen. Comp. Endocrinol., 25,* 126.

of islets of tissue surrounded by internal carotid vessels, capillaries of which interdigitate into the islets. The intermediate lobe surrounds the neurohypophysis ventrally.

Cytologically the gland contains large basophils in the rostral division of the pars distalis while the distal lobe proximal division is comprised largely of acidophils and the ventral lobe of mixed cell types. The pars intermedia contains one type of cell. The neurohypophysis is similar to that of elasmobranchs; there is a median eminence present and neurosecretory fibres running from the hypothalamus and interdigitating with the pars intermedia and a saccus vasculosus. This latter structure is, in *Latimeria*, incompletely separated from the posterior neurohypophysis. The presence of a median eminence appears to exclude any significant direct innervation of the pars distalis. A well-developed hypothalamo-hypophysial portal system is present. As there appears to be some direct connection between the neurohypophysis and the pars distalis then there may be a double innervation of the adenohypophysis in *Latimeria*. Nothing is known of the structure or function of coelocanth pituitary hormones.

The Dipnoii and the Actinopterygii

The bony fish pituitary is markedly different from that of the cyclostomes or elasmobranchs in that the neurohypophysis is in very close contact with all parts of the adenohypophysis. There is a well-developed saccus vasculosus in many species situated behind the pituitary but, as in other fish, although this latter structure arises from the infundibulum it has no endocrine function. Sometimes the saccus is absent, particularly in fresh water fish and in dipnoians.

The method of origin of the hypophysis in bony fish is by a solid ingrowth of ectoderm from under the forebrain. In a few fish a cavity may be formed which may persist as a hypophysial cavity in the adult. The hypophysis sinks in and attaches itself to the infundibulum but no infundibular stalk is developed. No lateral lobes develop but nervous tissue interdigitates completely into the adenohypophysis. Sometimes the adenohypophysis has a follicular structure, particularly in the rostral pars distalis region (Figure 1.12).

The adenohypophysis differentiates histologically, often very clearly, into three zones, the rostral pars distalis, the proximal pars distalis and the pars intermedia. These regions of the adenohypo-

Figure 1.12: Development of Trout Pituitary. Sagittal sections. (a) 7mm embryo. (b) 10mm embryo. (c) 65mm embryo. N, notochord; FG, foregut; FB, forebrain; H, hypophysis; ME, mouth epithelium; IC, infundibular cavity; SV, saccus vasculosus; PN, pars nervosa; PI, pars intermedia; PPD, proximal pars distalis; RPD, rostral pars distalis.

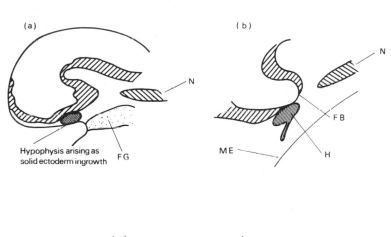

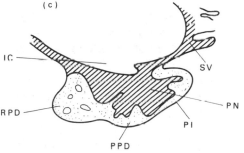

physis have been a source of nomenclature confusion for many years. The central proximal pars distalis was once regarded as a transitional area and called the 'ubergangsteil', while the rostral pars distalis was sometimes known as the pars tuberalis. In order to present neutral terms which implied no homology with the pituitary of other vertebrates the zones were called the pro-, meso- and meta-hypophysis. However, with advances in cytophysiology it became evident that a pars distalis and a pars intermedia do have a functional homology with these areas of higher vertebrate pituitaries. The division of the pars distalis is a matter of descriptive convenience but is useful in view of the often marked cytological difference between the rostral and proximal portion of the pars distalis. Until a more complete embryological survey is taken of fish pituitary and an attempt made to compare developmental histology with functional cytology and embryology in higher vertebrates then the terms rostral pars distalis, proximal pars distalis, pars intermedia and neurohypophysis should be used to designate parts of the actinopterygian pituitary. This convention also applies to the elasmobranch pituitary.

The Pituitary of Primitive Bony Fish

(a) The Dipnoi or lung fish probably arose from the ancestral fish stock at much the same time as the crossopterygians, that is, during the Lower Devonian period and although a number of families in this group of fish have become extinct two families still survive. These two families, the Ceratodontidae and the Lepidosirenidae comprise the lung fish of Australia, South America and Africa.

These animals, relatives of those animals which gave rise to the tetrapods, are particularly interesting in that their pituitaries resemble those of amphibians more closely than any other group of fish.

A mid-sagittal section through the pituitary of *Protopterus* reveals a structure very similar to that seen in urodele amphibian pituitary (Figure 1.13). There is a well-defined pars intermedia which is dorsal in position, a ventral pars distalis and a neurohypophysial cavity present but there is no saccus vasculosus. It is difficult to distinguish a proximal from a rostral pars distalis. The cytology of the pars distalis reveals three different types of basophils and at least two different forms of acidophils. These cells have variously been identified as possibly producing TSH, GH and gonadotropins but the evidence upon which this is based is equivocal. The pars intermedia consists of two types of cell, a PAS-positive basophil cell and a PAS-negative basophil cell. There is some evidence that, as in other fish, MSH is secreted by this part of the gland. Total hypophysectomy of the lungfish leads to melanin concentration while removal of the pars distalis alone

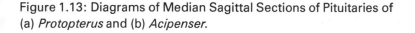

Figure 1.13: Diagrams of Median Sagittal Sections of Pituitaries of (a) *Protopterus* and (b) *Acipenser*.

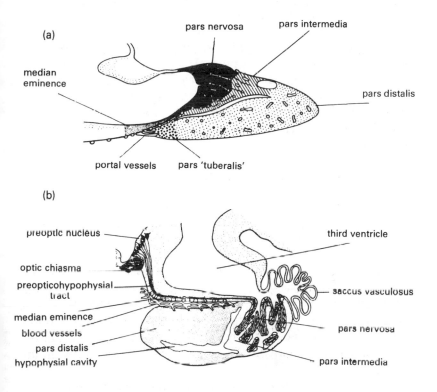

Source: (a) Based on Wingstrand, K.G. (1956) The structure of the pituitary in the African lung fish, *Protopterus annecteus* (Owen). *Videnskabelige Meddelelelser fra Dansk Naturhistorisk Forening i Kjøbenhaven*, 118, 193. (b) Based on Polenov, A.L. (1966) On the proximal neurosecretory contact region of the pre-optico-hypophysial system in Acipenseridae. *Dokl. Akad. Nank. SSSR, 169,* 1467.

causes melanin dispersion and hypertrophy of the pars intermedia.

A median eminence is present in the pituitary of lung fish which is quite distinct and lies just in front of the gland. Its capillary network is supplied with neurosecreting fibres arising from the nucleus preopticus, and portal vessels run from this blood plexus to supply the pars distalis. This pathway is very similar to the situation in amphibia.

The development of the neurohypophysis of dipnoians

resembles that of the pars nervosa of tetrapods rather than that of other fishes. In the adult much neurosecretory material is present and the nerve processes intertwine with the pars intermedia cells. Arginine vasotocin has been identified pharmacologically in lungfish as has mesotocin. Their function is unknown.

(b) The primitive fish which comprise the orders Polypteriformes, Acipenseriformes, Amiiformes and Lepisosteiformes, that is the bichirs, the sturgeons, bowfish and garfish, have pituitaries the structural features of which differentiate them from other bony fish. The major distinguishing feature is that like the elasmobranchs and dipnoians but unlike the teleosts, there is a median eminence. This portal system links the infundibular floor rich in neurosecretory terminations with the pars distalis capillaries, as in other vertebrate pituitaries where the structure is present.

Sometimes in the case of the sturgeon, *Acipenser* (Figure 1.13), a large hypophysial cavity characterises the gland whereas in the bichir, *Polypterus*, the base of Rathke's pouch is preserved in the adult as a duct from the roof of the mouth penetrating the pars distalis. The pituitary of all this group of primitive fishes is characterised by a well-developed saccus vasculosus which in the case of *Amia*, the bowfish, is very elongated. The rostral and proximal pars distalis and pars intermedia contain cells, basophils and acidophils, of the type seen in all other bony fish. The neurohypophysis penetrates into the pars intermedia but unlike the teleosts there is no penetration into the pars distalis.

The Pituitary of the Higher Actinopterygii (Teleostei)

The teleost pituitary differs from all other fish pituitaries in that the neurohypophysis ramifies into all regions of the adenohypophysis and in that there is no median eminence. It has been suggested that in this group the median eminence has become invaginated into the pars distalis and that blood from the capillaries surrounding the neurohypophysis supplies the pars distalis and pars intermedia with its equivalent of a portal flow. The pars distalis cells also appear to be directly innervated. The general ground plan of the teleost pituitary is seen in Figure 1.14.

Figure 1.14: Diagram to Illustrate the Main Features and the Blood Supply to the Cyprinodont Pituitary. Anterior to the left. (A) rostral pars distalis, (B) proximal pars distalis, and (C) pars intermedia. Neurohypophysial core (D). Blood enters the gland from the hypophysial artery (h), and passes to the primary longitudinal plexus (F) in the neurohypophysial core. From here it is distributed to the adenohypophysis in the secondary centrifugal plexus (E), and is then collected into a superficial venous network (black) (G) and passes to the hypophysial vein (j).

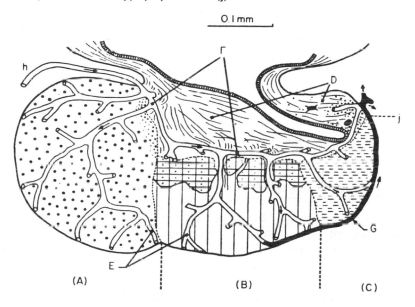

Source: Modified from Follenius (1965) by Ball, J.N. and Baber, B.I. (1969) The pituitary gland: anatomy and histopathology, in W.S. Hoar and D.J. Randall (eds.) *Fish Physiology*, vol. II. Academic Press, New York, pp. 1-110.

Cytology

The adenohypophysis of teleosts comprising rostral and proximal pars distalis and pars intermedia is composed of many different types of cells some of which have, with fair certainty, been identified with the production of specific hormones.

The rostral pars distalis is generally composed largely of acidophilic cells although in a number of species studied basophils also occur, as do chromophobic cells.

The acidophil cells, which in a number of species such as the eel are arranged in follicles, stain with a number of dyes such as erythrosin, Orange G, and azo-carmine but are not PAS positive. These cells have been identified as prolactin secreting. This identification comes about not only from cytophysiological evidence but also from the fact that these cells can demonstrate an immunofluorescent reaction to prolactin antibodies. Rabbit anti-sheep prolactin serum is prepared, fish pituitary sections incubated in it, and then 'stained' with a fluorescein-conjugated swine anti-rabbit globulin.

Between the groups of acidophilic cells lie small groups of basophils which are PAS positive and are in some species such as the eel regarded as TSH-secreting cells. These so-called thyrotrophs do not always occur in the rostral pars distalis but are found in the minnow and the roach in the proximal pars distalis and become degranulated and vacuolated when goitrogenic, drugs are introduced into fish.

The chromophobe cells of the rostral pars distalis are not always refractory to stain and in some species lead-haematoxylin staining clearly delineates these cells which often lie in the region between the prolactin cells and the neurohypophysis. Direct evidence for the ACTH secreting nature of these chromophobe cells has been obtained by treating fish with the drug metopirone (2-methyl-1-2-di-3'-pyridylpropan-1-one). This drug inhibits the 11-hydroxylation of adrenal steroids and by negative feedback results in hypertrophy of the chromophobe cells which can reasonably be expected, therefore, to be a source of ACTH.

The proximal pars distalis of teleosts consists generally of well-defined acidophils and basophils. The acidophils of this region are much more Orange G positive than those of the rostral pars distalis. They are PAS negative and generally coarsely granulated. Circumstantial evidence indicates that these cells are growth hormone producing and although these cells are now called somatotrophs the evidence that they do indeed produce somatotrophin is not overwhelming.

The PAS-positive basophils of the proximal pars distalis are variable in size and function. One type of basophil has finer granulation and is generally located dorsally in the region while another large basophil which often contains hyaline droplets is located ventrally. The more ventral basophils secrete the gonadotrophic hormone(s) while the more dorsal basophils produce the thyroid-stimulatory hormone. The evidence that these cells are indeed gonadotrophs and thyrotrophs is very convincing. The thyrotrophs which as has been previously mentioned also occur in some species in the rostral pars distalis, were shown in the minnow, *Phoxinus,* many years ago to respond to goitrogens by becoming hyper-trophied and vacuolated. This has been confirmed in many species of teleosts.

The gonadotrophs of teleosts have probably received more attention than any other cell of the fish pituitary. They have been shown to change in size and cellular content with age and repro-ductive condition, and after castration. Whether or not there are two types of gonadotroph cells, one of which secretes an LH-like hormone and the other an FSH-like hormone is not clear.

The pars intermedia is generally the most posterior of the adenohypophysial regions and shows much size variation in different species. In the salmonids it may form as much as two-thirds the volume of the pituitary. Two cell types are present except in salmonids where there is only one. Of these two cell types the staining is very variable but one is PAS positive and the other lead-haematoxylin positive. The PAS-positive cells may be basophilic, amphiphilic or acidophilic or absent in salmonids. The lead-haematoxylin cells appear to secrete the hormone MSH and, when viewed in electron micrographs, have a structure similar to mammalian MSH cells.

The neurohypophysis of teleosts is composed of hypothalamic neurosecretory fibres, glial cells and blood vessels. The nerve fibres are mainly non-myelinated and terminate in the central area of the neurohypophysis in close relationship to blood vessels. However, some fibres extend into the adenohypophysis and this inter-digitation particularly into the pars intermedia is, as has been men-tioned before, characteristic of the teleost pituitary. At least two types of neurohypophysial fibres can be distinguished, those which can be stained with neurosecretory stains and those which cannot. The stainable (Type A) fibres appear to originate from the nucleus preopticus of the hypothalamus whereas the non-stainable fibres originate from the nuclear lateralis tuberis. The blood capillaries of the neurohypophysis are covered with the termination of the neurocrine fibres as are many of the adenohypophysial cells. But the way in which these fibres innervate cells and transmit their secretory products to capillaries is complex and incompletely understood, and an equivalence of a median eminence, if one

exists, difficult to construct. The presence of the glial cells, or pitui-
cytes, adds further complications, for whereas in most vertebrates
these cells are regarded as essentially support cells, in teleosts they
may be directly involved in the functioning of the neurohypophysis. Some may transmit neurosecreting material from the axon
synapses into basement membranes, while others may be concerned with the autolysis of neurosecreting granules.

It is clear from the above description of the cytology of the teleost pituitary that numerous hormones are produced by this gland
and the biochemistry and physiological role of these hormones
must be described. As in all other groups of vertebrates the
removal of the gland has played an important part in this understanding. Removal of the pituitary was reported as early as 1911
by von Frisch in an investigation of pigment cells in fish and in fact
most of the experiments involving the removal of the pituitary for
the first 50 years of this century were concerned with either trying
to assess the role of the pituitary in colouration or reproduction in
teleosts. Hypophysectomy has helped to clarify the presence and
role of all the adenohypophysial hormones now known to be present in the teleost pituitary, namely growth hormones (GH),
thyroid stimulating hormone (TSH), gonadotropin, adrenocortico-
tropic hormone (ACTH), prolactin and the melanocyte-stimulating
hormone (MSH).

Hormones of the Adenohypophysis

Growth Hormone. Pickford in 1953 hypophysectomised male
killifish (*Fundulus heteroclitus*) and observed cessation of growth.
She then showed that hypophysectomised fish increased in length
when injected with mammalian growth hormone preparations.
Very few other teleosts have been hypophysectomised and growth
measured but both the swordtail (*Poecilia* sp.) and the rainbow
trout ceased to grow after pituitary removal. Growth hormone in
various degrees of purification has been obtained from the pituitaries of pollack (*Pollachius virens*), hake (*Urophycis tenuis*),
chinook salmon (*Oncorhynchus tshawytscha*) and *Tilapia* (*T.
mossambica*). The biochemical and fractionation procedures for
preparation have been based on those used to isolate mammalian
GH. *Tilapia* growth hormone has been shown to have biological
activity similar to that of NIH-GH-bovine growth hormone when
assayed for growth promotion in fish. *Tilapia* growth hormone has
also been shown by gel filtration to have a molecular weight of

22,000 which is very similar to that of the human GH monomer. The isoelectric point of fish growth hormone is similar to that of mammalian GH. The chemical characterisation of fish GH has been attempted and *Tilapia* GH resembles ovine GH in having two disulphides, a single tryptophan and low methionine and histidine content, but differs from ovine GH in having a high aspartic acid and serine content and a low alanine content. These differences in amino acid composition are reflected in biological activity. The growth hormone of teleosts is different from that of other vertebrates including other fishes. Growth hormone extracts from elasmobranchs, holosteans, dipnoi and chondricthyeans all give positive responses to the rat tibia growth assay but teleosts, with one exception, give no response. The highly purified *Tilapia* growth hormone mentioned above has been labelled with I^{125} and shown to bind specifically to liver membrane fractions of other teleosts. This binding affinity may form the basis of radioreceptor assay for teleost growth hormones. Although teleost GH does not promote growth in mammals, mammalian (and elasmobranch) growth hormone shows good growth promoting ability in teleosts (Table 1.2). If the condition factor (weight/length^3), an index of fatness or leanness of fish, is measured after growth hormone treatment it is found to be lowered indicating that the hormone promotes greater growth in length than weight.

Growth hormone appears to increase linear growth in fish in a number of ways. The hormone increases appetite, improves food

Table 1.2: Growth Hormone Activity of Pituitary Extracts and Growth Hormone Preparations from Various Vertebrate Sources in Various Groups of Vertebrates Excluding the Effects of Mammalian Growth Hormone Preparations in Mammals[a]

Growth bioassay	Source of pituitary extract or growth hormone preparation									
	Ag-natha	Elasmo-branch	Dip-noi	Chon-drostei	Holo-stei	Tele-ostei	Am-phibia	Rep-tilia	Aves	Mam-malia
Teleostei		+				+				+
Amphibia	−					−	+	+	+	+
Reptilia							±			+
Aves										+
Mammalia	−	+	+	+	−	+	+	+		
	+					+				

[a] +, positive effect; −, negative result.

Source: From Donaldson *et al.* (1979) in W.S. Hoar, D.J. Randall and Brett (eds.) *Fish Physiology*, vol. III. Academic Press, New York, p. 462.

conversion, increases protein synthesis, decreases nitrogen loss, stimulates fat mobilisation and oxidation, and stimulates either directly or indirectly insulin synthesis and release.

The increase in appetite in killifish and salmon which is evident after growth hormone treatment may be due to the growth hormone having a direct action on centres in the hypothalamus which influence food intake or the hormone may have an indirect effect on the hypothalamic centres by bringing about some metabolic changes in the fish. Improved food conversion, i.e. a decrease in the ratio of dry food or protein fed per gram gain in live weight, is in all probability due to changes in protein, fat or carbohydrate metabolism brought about by the hormone in a similar manner to that which occurs in mammals.

Castration of maturing Pacific salmon results in growth increase, which is correlated with hypertrophy and hyperplasia of the somatotrops of the proximal pars distalis. These somatotrops like the prolactin secretory cells of teleosts selectively locate the fluorescent antibody to mammalian growth hormone.

Prolactin. In mammals prolactin or the leutotropic hormone directs its action largely to the female. It acts synergistically with the luteinising hormone (LH), to develop and maintain a functional corpus luteum. It is responsible for the initiation of milk secretion in the mammary gland and in birds stimulates hyperplasia of epithelial cells of the crop gland to produce crop milk. With no receptors in fish similar to those in birds and mammals for prolactin the existence of a prolactin-like hormone in fish was for many years doubted, although a pigeon crop-stimulating factor had been claimed to exist in the teleost pituitary. Fish pituitary extracts were found to have no effect on mammary glands or crop sacs but it was shown by Grant and Pickford that fish pituitary extract was able to induce the return to water ('water drive') of hypophysectomised newts. This property was also shared by mammalian pituitary extracts and mammalian prolactin. These observations which showed for the first time that the fish pituitary possessed a factor that elicited a response in common with that of mammalian prolactin stimulated research in this direction. It has now been established that the teleost pituitary contains a factor which plays an important part in enabling fish to maintain their electrolyte and water balance in fresh water. Mammalian prolactin when injected into certain hypophysectomised euryhaline fish such as *Fundulus* and *Xiphophorus* enable the fish to survive in fresh water when normally they would need to be transferred to dilute (1:3) sea water in order to survive. Other fresh water teleosts though can survive in fresh water after hypophysectomy but electrolyte balance is impaired. For example in the eel *Anguilla anguilla* there is a slow reduction in plasma sodium and calcium after hypophysectomy. This fall can be prevented by therapy with mammalian prolactin. Again in brown trout hypophysectomy results in a decrease in water turnover which is corrected by prolactin treatment. There is thus no doubt that prolactin is a most important hydro-mineral regulating hormone in euryhaline fish.

The role of prolactin in sea-water teleosts is not so clearly defined as in freshwater, particularly euryhaline teleosts, although prolactin does seem to involve a reduction of the sodium efflux in several marine species. In the flounder, *Platichthys flescus*, prolactin reduces the sodium turnover by 50 per cent but sodium efflux is not significantly reduced in this species. Also in the starry flounder, *Platichthys stellatus*, prolactin reduced bladder water permeability and water permeability of the kidney tubules. Renal and gill sodium-potassium activated ATP-ase activity is also reduced by prolactin. Whether these effects in sea-water teleosts are physiological is uncertain.

Although prolactin modifies water and sodium movements through the gill, kidney and urinary bladder the hormone also affects the skin and gut. For example, prolactin lowers the water absorption from the sea-water-adapted eel and the stickleback and causes dispersal of xanthophore pigment in the skin of some fish such as gobies and pufferfish.

Prolactin has been shown to be involved in lipid metabolism and fat storage and also to reduce thyroxine levels of the serum.

The first highly purified prolactin was prepared from *Tilapia mossambica* and was shown to have a molecular weight of 19,400 and the amino acid composition revealed the presence of one tryptophan and four half-cystine residues which is characteristic of all known vertebrate growth hormones but not of mammalian prolactins. Tilapia prolactin has considerably more effect on teleost water and sodium retention than ovine prolactin but does not stimulate mammary tissue or the pigeon crop sac. Salmon (*Oncorhynchus keta*) prolactin has also been isolated and has been found to have more leucine and aspartic acid residues than other teleost prolactins (Table 1.3).

Table 1.3: Amino Acid Compositions of Flounder, Carp, Salmon, *Tilapia*, and Ovine Prolactin

Amino acid	Flounder	Carp	Salmon	*Tilapia*	Ovine
Lys	14.2	16.6	13.5	8.9	9
His	2.9	4.2	5.2	4.9	8
Arg	7.6	9.4	8.8	6.8	11
Asp	20.5	24.0	26.5	16.4	22
Thr	24.6	13.6	8.8	9.4	9
Ser	17.8	18.0	19.9	21.6	15
Glu	19.6	18.8	18.6	17.4	22
Pro	8.5	10.8	9.2	10.8	11
Gly	12.9	15.6	12.6	8.1	11
Ala	15.3	13.2	11.8	9.6	9
Half-Cys	3.4	5.0	3.4	4.2	6
Val	9.1	9.3	8.9	6.8	10
Met	3.3	4.6	4.7	5.4	7
Ile	8.5	5.5	8.1	9.3	11
Leu	16.9	17.6	26.2	24.5	23
Tyr	4.1	3.6	5.4	3.0	7
Phe	7.2	7.2	7.4	4.7	6
Trp	N.D.	N.D.	N.D.	1.0	2

N.D., Not determined.

Source: Idler, D.R. *et. al.* (1978) *Gen. Comp. Endocrinol., 35,* 409 and Ng, T.B. *et. al.* (1980) *Gen. Comp. Endocrinol., 42,* 141.

Levels of plasma prolactin are influenced both by light and temperature (Figure 1.15) and circadian rhythms in plasma prolactin have been seen in a number of species of teleost fish. These changes in levels have been suggested as being adaptive changes to temperature and light-induced activity; an increase of both would result in metabolic rate increase and increased sodium loss. Increased prolactin secretion may compensate for this loss. Similarly a decrease in metabolism may result in a decrease of prolactin secretion.

Thyrotropin. The teleost pituitary contains and releases a thyrotropic hormone (TSH) which regulates thyroid function. The hormone, a glycoprotein, has been purified and isolated. It has the same molecular weight as bovine TSH (28,000) and similar amino acid composition although eel TSH amino acid composition is less like bovine TSH in its amino acid composition than other mammalian TSHs such as mouse, sheep or man. Nevertheless the amino acid profiles of all teleost TSHs that have been isolated are generally similar.

Figure 1.15: Serum Prolactin Levels in *C. auratus* at 3-h Intervals over a 24-h Period. The ordinate is the concentration expressed as a percentage deviation from a reference standard. The abscissa is the time of day samples were taken and also represents the 16 h light : 8 h dark photoperiod, the clear area (light) is the photophase and the striped area (dark) is the scotophase. Each point represents the mean ± standard error for six samples. The solid line represents fish acclimated to 20°C and the broken line is for fish kept at 10°C.

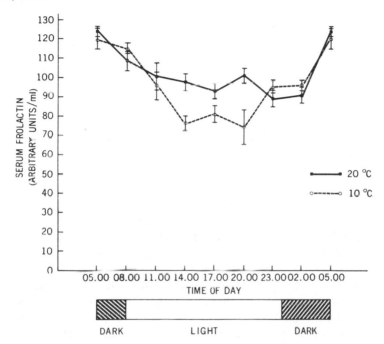

Source: McKeown, B.A., and Peter, R.E. (1976). The effects of photoperiod and temperature on the release of prolactin from the pituitary gland of the goldfish, *Carassius auratus* L. *Can. J. Zool.*, *54*, 1960-8.

Although both mammalian TSH and teleost TSH produce a linear log-dose response in fish thyroid cell height and hormone secretion teleost TSH is relatively inactive, or totally inactive on the mammalian thyroid. The teleost thyroid can also be stimulated by mammalian growth hormone. It appears that the teleost thyroid is poor at discriminating between mammalian growth hormone and mammalian TSH. Mammalian TSH is more active on starved trout or hypophysectomised eels at 20 or 25°C than at 10-15°C whereas carp TSH is equally active at both the higher and lower temperatures. Fish pituitaries contain variable amounts of TSH and this could, as will be seen in Chapter 2, relate to thyroid involvement in growth, reproduction or other metabolic activities. The pituitaries of some fish have a TSH content that may be 10-20 times as great as that found in mammals. The lungfish, *Protopterus annectens*, has a high pituitary content of TSH, and although thyroid activity in this fish is reduced during its period of activation no reduction in levels of pituitary TSH occur.

Adrenocorticotropin (ACTH). ACTH has been shown to be present in the anterior pituitary of many teleosts and its release controlled through negative feedback with the adrenocorticosteroids. This hormone is distinct from the melanocyte stimulating hormone which has a similar amino acid composition. In the salmon specific cells (the corticotrops) localise fluorescent-labelled antibodies to porcine ACTH and synthetic ACTH. This indicates a structural similarity between mammalian and teleost ACTH. Mammalian ACTH stimulates the production of teleost adrenal steroids. Also teleost ACTH stimulates the production of mammalian adrenal steroids. Partially purified Pacific salmon ACTH causes increase in cortisol levels in trout and this response is similar to that obtained by porcine ACTH.

Melanophore Stimulating Hormone (MSH). Colour change in cyclostomes and elasmobranchs, i.e. dispersion or contraction of the pigment granules of the dermal chromatophores, is regulated by means of MSH. However, in the teleosts colour response is in part controlled by the sympathetic nervous system and it has long been known that the melanophores of teleosts are innervated. Colour change in teleosts is, though, also regulated by a melanophore stimulating hormone. Perfusion of an eel skin with teleost pituitary extract can cause dispersion of pigment granules of chromatophores in a matter of minutes. If, though, an eel is taken from a black background and placed on a white background, or hypophysectomised, maximum pallor does not develop for many days. The response to endogenous MSH is a slow one but nevertheless there does appear to be a hormonal control of pigment dispersion.

Some teleosts appear to be little affected by MSH. Injection of Fundulus, the killifish, or the minnow (*Phoxinus phoxinus*) pituitary into the same species has variable or little effect on colour. Also in these species hypophysectomy does not introduce a permanent state of pallor as it does in the eel. It is known in these species that the melanophores are innervated by pigment aggregating fibres and it may be that the influence of these fibres overrides the hormonal pigment dispersing effect. Attempts have been made to identify a melanin concentrating hormone in the pituitary of teleosts but without result. For, as mentioned previously, many groups of teleosts contain two distinct types of cells in the pars intermedia but only one of these, the lead-haematoxylin, type I MSH secreting cell, shows hypertrophy when the animal is adapted to a black background. Placing the fish on a white background does not induce hypertrophy of any pars intermedia cell.

The primary structure of teleost MSH has only recently been elucidated although some years ago cod (*Gadus*) pituitary was subject to starch-gel electrophoresis and two components migrating to similar positions as mammalian α-MSH and mammalian β-MSH were identified. Both α- and β-MSH have been isolated in the salmon *Oncorhynchus keta* (Figure 1.16). The α-MSH is identical to mammalian α-MSH except for an unacelylated *N*-terminus. β-MSH is very similar to that of mammals.

Gonadotropic Hormone(s) (GTH). It has been known for many years that the pituitary of bony fishes secretes one or more gonadotropic hormones. Many experiments involving injection of pituitary gland extracts and implantation and ablation of the gland correlated with gonadal changes have established the presence of such a hormone(s). As mentioned previously GTH originates in specific glycoprotein-containing cells of the pars distalis but whether or not there are two distinct types of cell producing an 'LH' and an 'FSH' form of hormone is problematic. Experimental immunocytological and electron microscope studies have failed to demonstrate two types of gonadotropic cell in the Atlantic salmon, *Salmo salar*, but on the other hand two different types of gonadotrophs are claimed to be present in the Masu salmon, *Oncorhynchus masou*, the white-spotted char, *Salvelinus leucomaenis* and in the loach, *Misgurnus anguillacaudatus*.

The earliest attempt to isolate and purify teleost GTH was made by Otsuka in 1956. He, and subsequently other workers, were able

Figure 1.16: Sequence Comparison of Melanotropins from Various Vertebrates. (G): a gap in amino acid sequence.

α-MSH
```
salmon    H-Ser-Tyr-Ser-Met-Glu-His-Phe-Arg-Trp-Gly-Lys-Pro-Val-NH2
dogfish   H-Ser-Tyr-Ser-Met-Glu-His-Phe-Arg-Trp-Gly-Lys-Pro-Met-NH2/OH
mammals   CH3CO- Ser-Tyr-Ser-Met-Glu-His-Phe-Arg-Trp-Gly-Lys-Pro-Val-NH2
```

β-MSH
```
salmon    H-Asp-Gly-(G)-Ser-Tyr-Lys-Met-Asn-His-Phe-Arg-Trp-Ser-Gly-Pro-Pro-Ala-Ser-OH
dogfish   H-Asp-Gly-Ile-Asp-Tyr-Lys-Met-Gly-His-Phe-Arg-Trp-Gly-Ala-Pro-Met-Asp-Lys-OH
dogfish   H-Asp-Gly-Asp-Asp-Tyr-Lys-Phe-Gly-His-Phe-Arg-Trp-Ser-Val-Pro-Leu-OH
macacus   H-Asp-Glu-Gly-Pro-Tyr-Arg-Met-Glu-His-Phe-Arg-Trp-Gly-Ser-Pro-Pro-Lys-Asp-OH
porcine   H-Asp-Glu-Gly-Pro-Tyr-Lys-Met-Glu-His-Phe-Arg-Trp-Gly-Ser-Pro-Pro-Lys-Asp-OH
equine    H-Asp-Glu-Gly-Pro-Tyr-Lys-Met-Glu-His-Phe-Arg-Trp-Gly-Ser-Pro-Arg-Lys-Asp-OH
bovine    H-Asp-Ser-Gly-Pro-Tyr-Lys-Met-Glu-His-Phe-Arg-Trp-Gly-Ser-Pro-Pro-Lys-Asp-OH
camel     H-Asp-Gly-Gly-Pro-Tyr-Lys-Met-Gln-His-Phe-Arg-Trp-Gly-Ser-Pro-Pro-Lys-Asp-OH
camel     H-Asp-Gly-Gly-Pro-Tyr-Lys-Met-Glu-His-Phe-Arg-Trp-Gly-Ser-Pro-Pro-Lys-Asp-OH
```

Source: Kawauchi, H., and Muramoto, K. (1979). Isolation and primary structure of melanotropins from salmon pituitary glands. *Int. J. Peptide Protein Res., 14*, 373-4.

to show that ethanol and acetone acetic acid extracts caused testis growth both in mice and trout and spermiation in the frog. Since then numerous preparations from several fish have been isolated and shown to have high gonadotropic activity. However, incomplete purification coupled with the use of non-fish bioassays have made it difficult to assess the number of gonadotropins in the fish pituitary. The weight of evidence now appears to favour the presence of multiple gonadotropins. These may be divided up into those gonadotropins which are rich in carbohydrates and those which are poor in carbohydrates. The carbohydrate-rich gonadotropins are possibly involved in such processes as steroidogenesis, spermiation, oocyte maturation and ovulation while the carbohydrate-poor gonadotropins may be physiologically more concerned with vitellogenesis, i.e. the production of egg yolk. However, carbohydrate-rich gonadotropins have been shown in some species to stimulate vitellogenesis. Sexual differences may also occur in gonadotropin biochemistry.

In spite of the biochemical and biological difficulties of isolating fish gonadotropins a number of radioimmunoassays have been developed for these hormones. This has enabled an indication to be given of hormonal changes, both in the pituitary and in the plasma, that are associated with reproduction. Increased plasma titres occur with maturity, both in male and female salmonids. The majority of studies though have not detected any changes in plasma gonadotropins during the early stages of gonadal development.

There is good evidence for gonadal regulation of gonadotropic function in teleosts. After castration of the mature rainbow trout gonadotropin secretion increases but as one might expect the response varies with the season in which the operation is performed. Changes in gonadotropic cells have also been observed to occur in the pituitary of Pacific salmon after castration.

Synthetic LH-releasing hormone when injected into teleosts brings about an increase in plasma GTH (Figure 1.17). Probably the major factors acting upon gonadotropin release in fish, via hypothalamic releasing factors, are environmental. Levels of gonadotropins have been shown to change in direct response to temperature and light. Salmonids are more responsive to changes in photoperiodicity while cyprinids are more responsive to changes in temperature. However, such generalisations should be made with caution for the integration and mutual dependence of these two environmental cues to GTH secretion and hence spawning are complex. In the rainbow trout gonadotropin appears to have short-term bursts of secretion during the day and night but these are not synchronised to the diurnal light cycle; individual fish have individual rhythms.

Hypothalamic Release Hormones. Hypothalamic control of pituitary gland secretion in fishes conforms to the general vertebrate pattern and the number of factors and peptides isolated from the brain of fish influencing pituitary function mirrors those found in mammals. Few experiments have been made in fish, however, in which lesions or electrical stimulation of the hypothalamus has

Figure 1.17: Plasma GTH and 17β-E$_2$ Profiles after Two Injections of LH-RH (3 μg/kg Body Weight) in 5 Female Z-strain Carp. First injection at 0 h, second injection 3 h later. Blood samples were taken at 0, 1/2, 1, 3, 3 1/2, 5, 7, 9 and 12 h. Basic level: GTH and 17β-E$_2$ levels at 0 h. Each point represents the mean, the vertical lines the standard deviations. Differences between values are expressed as: NS = non-significant, $*P < 0.05$, $**P < 0.01$, $***P < 0.005$.

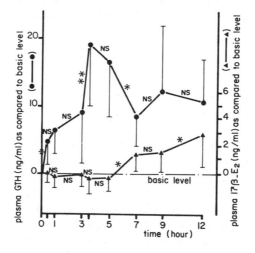

Source: Weil, C. *et. al.* (1980). Profiles of plasma gonadotropin and 17β-estradiol in the common carp, *Cyprinus carpio* L., as related to spawning induced by hypophysation or LH-RH treatment. *Reprod. Nutr. Dévelop., 20 (4A)*, 1041-50.

resulted in gonadal, adrenocortical or thyroid secretion. The approach in fish has been to inject mammalian release or inhibitory factor as they have been available in a purified state and to observe physiological effects or to assay brain material when a mammalian RIA has been developed. As the anatomical relationship between the brain and pituitary, particularly in respect to the blood supply for the brain of the latter, varies a great deal from one group of fish to another it would not be surprising if hormone release mechanisms differed widely.

Thyrotropin-Releasing Hormone (TRH). This hormone, a tri-peptide, has been isolated from the hypothalami of a number of mammalian species and has been shown to initiate TSH release (assayed by release of ^{131}I from thyroids of ^{131}I-treated rats), and in some mammals prolactin release. TRH has been identified in the brain of cyclostomes and teleosts using a radioimmunoassay for synthetic TRH. Synthetic TRH has no effect on the pituitary and thyroid cytology of cyclostomes but in some teleosts there is evidence that TRH inhibits iodine uptake by the thyroid. The administration of goldfish hypothalamic extracts decreases ^{131}I uptake by their thyroids. However, if synthetic TRH is injected by an intra-ventricular route then no changes in peripheral thyroxine levels are seen. At the present time it would seem that the release of TSH is controlled in teleosts by a manner not comparable to that of mammals.

Gonadotropin Releasing Hormone. A single decapeptide has been isolated in mammals which elicits the secretion of both luteinising hormone and follicle stimulating hormone. The peptide has been synthesised and a considerable number of analogues produced which show FSH or LH secretion stimulating activity.

Radioimmunoassay evidence for the presence of a gonado-tropin releasing hormone in the cyclostome brain is lacking but using an immunocytochemical unlabelled antibody enzyme technique mammalian-like immunoreactive material has been detected. Specific immunocytochemical staining is located in the pre-optic nuclei of lampreys and is very heavy in reproductive adults. However, in hagfish no immunocytochemical reaction can be detected and it may be that in this group of cyclostomes there is a degeneration of hypophysial-gonadal integration that occurs in all other vertebrates including lampreys.

In teleosts homologous radioimmunoassays for gonadotropin, as we have seen, have been developed and these have enabled the direct assay of brain extracts. Hypothalamic extracts of carp brain evoke a dose-related response of gonadotropin secretion by the carp pituitary both *in vitro* and *in vivo*. Crim and his co-workers using a radioimmunoassay for carp gonadotropin have shown that an intraventricular injection of hypothalamic extract or synthetic gonadotropin release hormone brings about comparable stimulations of hormone release in the goldfish while other brain regions extracted and tested were ineffective. Immature trout are unresponsive to synthetic-gonadotropin releasing hormone. Hypophysiotropic activity has thus been established for teleosts — a gonadotropin release factor — but its chemical composition and similarity to the mammalian decapeptide have yet to be established. Immunofluorescent studies have localised GRH in the forebrain and neurohypophysis of trout.

Growth Hormone Control

In mammals growth hormone secretion appears to be regulated by both a release and an inhibitory factor which act in concert with catecholamines, plasma carbohydrate, amino acid and lipid levels and stress. The growth process in vertebrates is a complicated story and fish are no exception to this story. A growth hormone release hypothalamic decapeptide has been isolated in mammals but its true role in growth has not yet been established. For example, it is capable of the release of bioassayable but not immunoassayable growth hormone. Also, in the mammalian hypothalamus a growth hormone release inhibitory factor has been isolated and is now known as 'somatostatin'. Somatostatin is a tetradecapeptide and inhibits growth hormone secretion from the pituitary of mammals both *in vivo* and *in vitro* and also inhibits TSH secretion.

There is no evidence of a growth hormone release factor in fish but somatostatin has been demonstrated by radioimmunoassay to be present in the brain of cyclostomes, chondrichthians and bony fish. Furthermore immunocytochemical identification of this factor in fish has permitted localisation of its distribution in the brain. Although somatostatin is present in fish its action on fish growth hormone release has not been fully established. This is largely because there exists for fish no homologous radioimmunoassay for growth hormone or sensitive quantitative bioassays. However, recently the pituitary glands of *Tilapia* have been incubated in synthetic somatostatin and by using a specific homologous radio-receptor assay it has been shown that growth hormone secretion is inhibited. Also the effect of somatostatin on TSH release has not been clearly established in fish.

In fish as in higher vertebrates somatostatin has been found distributed in tissues other than the hypothalamus. It is found for example throughout the brain of dogfish and ratfish and in the pancreas of cyclostomes and teleosts. The gastrointestinal and pancreatic distribution and function of somatostatin will be described in Chapter 00.

Several other hypothalamic releasing hormones have been identified in mammals, e.g. a corticotropin releasing hormone, but at present we cannot say if they exist in fish. The only unequivocal hypophysial-anterior pituitary link in fish is that of gonadotropin regulation although lesions of the hypothalamus increase thyroid activity in goldfish. In regulation of growth hormone release in mammals, catecholamines play a part, as mentioned above. Also in fish brain amines may play a role in pituitary hormone release but evidence thus far is scanty. MSH release appears to be under aminergic control for reserpine causes depletion of granules from the MSH cells and dispersion of the melanophores in the eel. However, 6-hydroxydopamine has been shown to destroy the aminergic neurosecretory fibres entering the rostral pars distalis of *Tilapia mossambica* but to have no effect on prolactin or ACTH release in this fish. Also whereas dopamine inhibits the release of growth hormone from incubated *Poecilia latipinna* pituitaries, this effect is not reversed by alpha or beta adrenergic antagonists such as phentolamine or propanolol.

Endorphins, i.e. opiate peptides, have been visualised immuno-cytochemically in the teleost hypothalamus and identified bio-chemically in the salmon pituitary. There is no evidence for any physiological role of these peptides in fish.

The Neurohypophysial Hormones of the Osteichthyes

The presence of the neurohypophysial peptides, arginine vaso-tocin, glumitocin, valiotocin and aspartocin in cyclostomes and elasmobranchs has already been mentioned and two other peptides *mesotocin* and *isotocin* have been identified in lungfish and the ray-finned fish. In total in all vertebrates nine active neurohypo-physial peptides have been identified, seven of them in fishes (Table 1.1). One group of these peptides contains basic amino acids in the 8 position of the peptide and the other group contains 'neutral' amino acids in this position. The first group is associated more with antidiuretic vasopressor pharmacological principles and the second group with oxytocin-like principles.

The peptide arginine vasotocin is found in all fishes and indeed in all vertebrates and it does appear perhaps to be the ancestral neurophysial principle from which all others have evolved. Considerable pharmacological investigations have been done on this peptide as they have on all naturally occurring neurohypophysial peptides. However, neither AVT nor the other peptides identified in all groups of fish have been identified with any definitive physiological role. Smooth muscle in fish, as in other vertebrates, is very sensitive to neurohypophysial peptides and this has given rise to the suggestion that the site of action of these principles may be on the oviduct. The oviduct smooth muscle preparation of certain poecilids will respond *in vitro* to picogram per millilitre quantities of AVT and the response is modified by oestrogen and gonadotropin. There is an indication then that the function of reproductive structures may be modulated by this peptide. It is, however, probably its effect on vascular smooth muscle that is more fundamental for fish and all vertebrate cardiovascular systems respond to neurohypophysial hormones in some manner. Isotocin and mesotocin (and oxytocin) constrict the branchial vessels and induce a reflex vasodilatation in the systemic vasculature. Arginine vasotocin is pressor in its effect and acts mainly on peripheral resistance. The threshold dose of AVT in the eel is about 5×10^{-11} mol kg^{-1}. In the same animal the threshold of isotocin required to raise the blood pressure is about 1×10^{-11} mol kg^{-1}.

Many experiments have been carried out in teleosts to establish a water balance and ion-regulatory role for neurohypophysial hormones. There appears to be no consistent effects and changes in water flow may result from capillary smooth muscle concentration. Neurohypophysial hormones may have an effect on the kidney glomeruli.

Metabolic roles for neurohypophysial hormones in fish have not been greatly explored. AVT injection in coho salmon fry increases plasma free fatty acids when administered in low concentrations, but decreases levels at higher concentrations. AVT also has been shown to increase levels of plasma glucose in salmon as it does in lampreys. Growth hormone in the blood is also increased by AVT.

Certain cyprinodont fish, for example the killifish *Fundulus heteroclitus*, exhibit a characteristic spawning behaviour in which

S-shaped flexure of the body occurs. This spawning reflex response can be elicited in individual isolated fish irrespective of sex by injection of neurohypophysial hormones. These injections are equally effective after hypophysectomy and castration. However the doses required are pharmacologically high suggesting that the response may be evoked by a non-physiological local stimulation of some brain centre.

It is disappointing that in spite of the large amount of pharmacological investigation, peptide biochemistry and elegant hypotheses of their molecular evolution we should know so little of the endocrine function of neurohypophysial hormones in teleosts and fish in general.

2 THE THYROID GLAND

The thyroid gland of cyclostomes and fishes shares two characteristics with the glands of all other vertebrates, first, its basic histological unit is a single cell walled follicle, and secondly this tissue is
capable of most efficiently trapping inorganic iodine and incor-
porating it into thyroid hormones. In this group of vertebrates the
follicles generally contain a central cavity filled with the glycoprotein secretion thyroglobulin but except in the elasmobranchs
and in a few teleosts the follicles are not aggregated together to
form a discrete and compact thyroid gland as is seen in the tetrapods.

In the adult lampreys the follicles are scattered in small groups
embedded in fibrous tissue along the floor of the pharynx, adjacent
to the ventral aorta. In the adult hagfish the thyroid follicles are
found isolated or in small groups embedded in the fatty tissue of
the pharyngeal wall along the course of the ventral aorta and as far
caudal as the last branchial sac. Whereas, the follicle diameters of
the adult lampreys are much the same, the size of the hagfish follicles
varies enormously within an individual animal (some may even
reach 2mm in diameter) although larger follicles occur with
increased frequency in larger animals. Also the follicles contain not
colloid-like secretory material occupying much of the central
cavity but coarsely granular material lying scattered in a largely
empty lumen. The hagfish thyroid epithelial cell structure also
differs from that of the typical thyroid epithelial cell in that it contains large inclusion bodies. The lamprey follicular colloid is more
typical of the vertebrate form and in general stains with aniline
blue, and is PAS positive. This material is possibly retained
colloid-like material.

The adult lamprey follicle epithelium has been distinguished
into three cell types one of which is ciliated. It is thought, though,
that these are different functional stages of the same cell type for
they all have the same electron micrographic structure. Large
yellow inclusions are also found in lamprey follicle epithelial cells
and are thought to be lysosomes.

Lampreys start life as an ammocoete larva and these larvae
undergo a metamorphosis to give the adult stage. In the larval

pharynx there is a structure known as the endostyle which gives rise to the thyroid gland at metamorphosis. The endostyle is formed from a sac, derived from and lying below the pharynx. This sac known as the subpharyngeal gland divides to form a pair of tubes, and within these tubes four rows of glandular cells develop. These rows of cells, which as the larvae develops coil to attain a relatively complex form, are of different types, some ciliated and some not. An opening is retained with the pharynx (Figure 2.1). Although this structure resembles the endostyle of *Amphioxus* its role in filter feeding is uncertain although it does secrete mucus in which food particles become entangled. It is, however, the structure which gives rise to the thyroid of the adult lamprey, the rows of epithelial cells transforming into thyroid follicles. The details of which cells of the endostyle complex form the epithelial cells of the adult follicle cells is unclear.

Figure 2.1: Cross-section through Endostyle of an Ammocoete Larva of a Lamprey. G, gill; P, pharynx; PBG, pseudobranchial groove; A, artery; L, lumen of endostyle; D, duct joining lumen to pharynx at one point; CE, ciliated epithelium; GE, glandular epithelium.

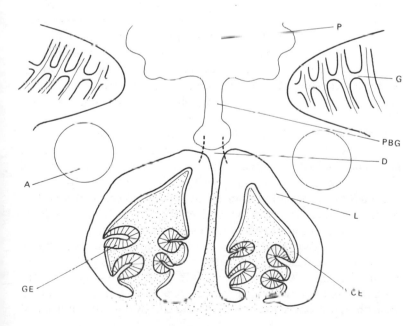

The interesting feature of this gland is not only that it develops into the thyroid but that it is capable of trapping iodine and synthesising the two thyroid hormones, 3, 5, 3' — triiodothyronine and thyroxine together with their precursors 3-monoiodotyrosine and 3, 5-diiodotyrosine. The endostyle is capable of this synthesis during the whole of larval life which may be five or six years. The two hormones bind to a protein in the endostyle and ultimately are released and find their way into the blood circulation. The concentrations of thyroxine in the serum of *Petromyzon marinus* larvae are high (ca. 8.0 µg/100ml) compared with that of the adult.

Although the lamprey endostyle produces thyroid hormones it is an 'exocrine' gland and not endocrine. This prompts the question — is there a feedback relationship between the pituitary gland and the endostyle of larval lampreys? Treatment with goitrogens such as thiourea or thiouracil which in tetrapods inhibit thyroidal biosynthesis and cause hypertrophy and hyperplasia of the gland results in marked changes in the ammocoete endostyle, the glandular tracts undergoing hypertrophy and hypervascularisation. This may not, however, be a result of TSH release as thyroxine does not produce any obvious alteration of the effect of thiourea when the two are administered together. Nevertheless injection of mammalian TSH into lamprey larvae results in hypertrophy of certain of the endostyle cells and an increase in iodine uptake. There is no evidence, as has been mentioned in Chapter 1, that TSH is produced by the ammocoete larva. Hypophysectomy does not result in cellular changes in the endostyle and strangely does not prevent the hypersecretory response to thiourea.

The development of the thyroid follicles in the embryo of hagfish is poorly understood. Our knowledge is dependent on a report from the beginning of the century in which the primordium of the thyroid is said to arise in the hagfish *Eptatretus stouti* by separation along most of the length of the median pharyngeal floor. The elongated primordium parts from the pharynx in the form of a continuous chain of cellular groups varying from one to as many as ten or more cells per group. The larger of these groups breaks down into smaller groups from which follicles arise.

The hormone thyroxine has been measured in the plasma of both hagfish and lamprey adults. In hagfish thyroxine levels are around 3.5 µg/100 ml plasma while that of lampreys is much lower, around 0.5 µg/100ml plasma. Attempts have been made to see if this hormone varies in concentration during metamorphosis and migration. As already mentioned the concentrations of thyroxine in the ammocoete larvae is high both in feeding and non-feeding larvae, and declines during metamorphosis. There is no evidence that thyroxine is in any way related to metamorphosis as it is in the amphibia. Also the evidence for an endogenous TSH in adult cyclostomes is equivocal.

The physiological role of the thyroid in hagfish and lampreys is virtually unknown. Some efforts have been made to correlate thyroid activity with spawning and reproduction but with no clear cut results. The iodine uptake of the river lamprey decreases when the animal is left in fresh water after capture. Other investigations have looked at various biochemical changes after injecting thyroid hormones. An increase in plasma free fatty acids, a decrease in plasma glucose and an increase in nitrogen retention have been observed, but all these changes may well be pharmacological ones.

The thyroid gland of chondrichthian fish is discrete and pear-shaped in sharks and dogfish and somewhat flattened and disc-shaped in skates and rays. The embryological origin of the gland is indicated by the fact that the narrow part of the shark thyroid is directed towards the pharyngeal floor. Indeed in one primitive shark (*Chlamydoselachus*) a duct extends from the narrow end of the thyroid through the basihyal cartilage to the pharynx.

The thyroid follicle of elasmobranchs is similar in structure to that found in bony fish and tetrapods. The follicle cells are normally cuboidal in shape but in the smaller follicles the cells are columnar. There is considerable variation in follicle diameter, and larger follicles are found in older animals. Large follicle shape varies filling into the shape of neighbouring follicles. Nuclei of the epithelial cells are basal and the cytoplasm is generally full of red granules and globules. Pycnotic nuclei are frequently found, and sometimes these pycnotic epithelial cells are found in the colloid of the follicles. The follicular colloid unlike that of cyclostomes is dense, eosinophilic and is not greatly vacuolated at its edge.

Although as has been previously mentioned TSH appears to be produced by the ventral lobe of the elasmobranch pituitary in that there is an increase of thyroxine release from thyroid glands of sharks incubated with ventral lobe homogenates there is no response of the thyroid when incubated with mammalian TSH. Thus it seems that the elasmobranch thyroid is highly specific in its response to elasmobranch TSH. Possibly this response is due to a specific amino acid sequence of the elasmobranch TSH.

Although TSH appears to be present in the elasmobranch pituitary its functional significance is uncertain for a thyroid - pituitary axis has as yet not been established. Hypophysectomy of the dogfish, *Scyliorhinus canicula* does not result in any histological changes in the thyroid but if embryos are decapitated the thyroid fails to complete its differentiation. The removal of the ventral pituitary lobe has not yet been accomplished. Also the goitrogens phenylthiourea or thiourea do not cause histological changes in the gland of rays or sharks.

Over 30 years ago, using radioactive ^{131}I, it was shown that thyroxine is synthesised in the dogfish thyroid in a manner similar to that in mammals, with monoiodotyrosine and diiodotyrosine being produced as precursors to thyroxine (Figure 2.2). The excretion of ^{131}I is rapid in elasmobranchs and takes place possibly largely through the gills as well as the usual biliary route.

In mammals the calorigenic effect of thyroid hormones is well known and it was therefore natural that, when the function of the elasmobranch (and bony fish) thyroid came to be examined, an attempt should be made to investigate the effect of elasmobranch thyroid hormone on oxygen consumption. Surgical thyroidectomy, however, had no significant effect on oxygen consumption. A transient effect of the thyroxine analogue, triiodothyroacetic acid on dogfish embryo oxygen uptake has been reported, but this is probably a pharmacological effect. Extracts of dogfish thyroid do, however, increase the oxygen consumption of rats. In spite of no demonstrable calorigenic effect dogfish liver mitochondria swell in the presence of thyroxine in much the same manner as mammalian liver mitochondria (Figure 2.3).

Early observations on the thyroid of dogfish clearly indicated that the thyroids of mature female dogfish were two or three times as large as those of mature males of comparable size. This sex difference led to attempts to relate thyroid gland activity with events in the sexual cycle and maturation of gonads. In the oviparous dogfish, *Scyliorhynus canicula*, thyroid activity (judged by histological criteria) is greatest in the male when the testes first become mature and in the female when the oocytes commence their first rapid growth. Also in ovoviviparous elasmobranchs hyperactivity of the thyroid is associated with gestation; and after parturition the glands return to an appearance of lower activity. Although this histological correlation undoubtedly exists between thyroid activity and gonadal development further hormonal

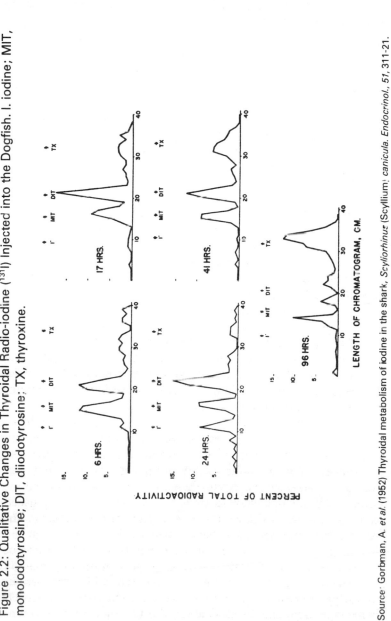

Figure 2.2: Qualitative Changes in Thyroidal Radio-iodine (¹³¹I) Injected into the Dogfish. I. iodine; MIT, monoiodotyrosine; DIT, diiodotyrosine; TX, thyroxine.

Source: Gorbman, A. *et al.* (1952) Thyroidal metabolism of iodine in the shark, *Scyliorhinus* (Scyllium) *canicula. Endocrinol., 51,* 311-21.

Figure 2.3: Kinetics of Swelling in 0.15 *M* KCl Solution of Dogfish Liver Mitochondria isolated in 0.44 *M* Sucrose and Incubated at 30°C. Compounds tested were present at 5×10^{-5} *M* concentration; mitochondrial protein, 0.5 mg per millilitre.

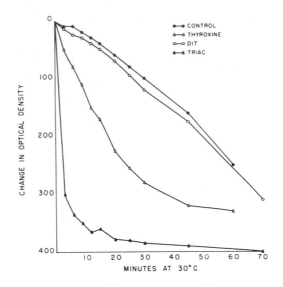

Source: Greif, R.L. and Alfano, J.A. (1964) Thyroid hormone induced swelling of isolated dogfish liver mitochondria. *Gen. Comp. Endocrinol., 4,* 339-42.

measurements need to be made in order to establish cause and effects. Do thyroid hormone titres rise in the blood before those of oestrogen and androgen or vice-versa?

Changes have been correlated between elasmobranch thyroid activity and migrating and seasonal variation and this phenomenon is discussed in Chapter 8. This correlation has also prompted investigation into the effect of thyroid hormones on osmoregulation in elasmobranchs. Osmoregulation is achieved in elasmobranchs by a controlled degree of uraemia and it is usually assumed that these fish do not face any serious problems in controlling water balance. However, in view of the known implication of the thyroid hormones in nitrogen metabolism in other vertebrates it is of interest to know whether these hormones play any part in the regulation of urea levels. Thyroidectomy of the euryhaline elasmobranch *Dasyatis sabina* results in a marked elevation of plasma urea levels (Table 2.1). Plasma osmotic levels are

Table 2.1: Changes in Plasma Solute Concentrations in Thyroidectomised[a] *Dasyatis sabina*

	Plasma Osmotic Concentration mOsm/l ($\overline{X}\pm$S.E.)	Urea mM/l ($\overline{X}\pm$S.E.)	Na+	Plasma K+ mEq/l ($\overline{X}\pm$S.E.)	Ca²⁺	Cl
(Medium Concentration — 840 mOsm/l						
Thyroidectomised (7)	1075±7[b]	464±7[b]	291±3	3.2±0.1	4.2±0.2	317±6
Sham operated (6)	1006±8	409±9	290±3	3.3±0.1	4.2±0.2	301±9
(Medium Concentration — 830 mOsm/l)						
Thyroidectomised (7)	1083±10[c]	454±13[b]	309±3[b]	3.6±0.2	3.2±0.2[b]	320±7
Sham operated (5)	1050±4	406± 5	319±2	3.8±0.2	4.3±0.1	323±5

[a]Sacrificed 10 days after thyroid removal.
[b]Significantly different ($P < 0.01$) than sham.
[c]Significantly different ($P < 0.05$) than sham.

Source: de Vlaming, V.L., Sage, M. and Beitz, B. (1975) Pituitary, adrenal and thyroid influences on osmoregulation in the euryhaline elasmobranch, *Dasyatis sabina. Comp. Biochem. Physiol., 52A*, 505-13.

also elevated but muscle water content and body weight loss are not affected thus the results are not due to a single change in plasma volume. However, whether thyroid hormone increases urea efflux or modifies urea metabolism is not clear.

The thyroid gland of bony fish, particularly the teleosts, has been intensively studied. But while the structure of the gland and the processes of synthesis of the thyroid hormone are well defined and are essentially the same as that in higher vertebrates the function of the gland remains somewhat enigmatic although recent researchers point to some very specific physiological roles.

The thyroid of most bony fish consists of isolated follicles scattered around the ventral aorta and its branches into the gills. This pattern of scattered follicles can extend quite widely outside the pharyngeal region. In some fish, for example the platyfish, follicles are found in the eye, kidney and other organs (Figure 2.4). This migration of so-called heterotropic follicles from the pharyngeal region is probably due to the fact that the gland is not encapsulated and surrounded by connective tissue. Some teleosts do though have an encapsulated thyroid, for example, parrot fish, sword fish and tuna. The encapsulated thyroid is provided with a good blood supply. Both the unencapsulated and encapsulated thyroid have characteristic follicles filled with 'colloid'.

Figure 2.4: Diagram of the Head Region of a Platyfish Showing
Distribution of Normal and Abnormal Thyroid Follicles.

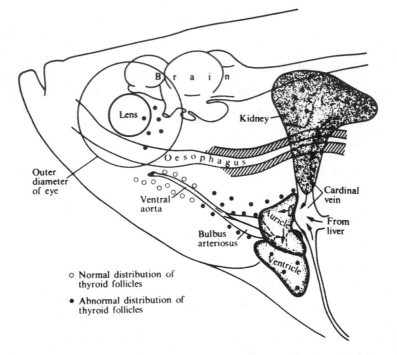

Source: Baker, K.F. *et al.* (1955) Functional thyroid tumours in the kidneys of platyfish.
Cancer Res., *15*, 118.

The epithelial cell may range from a flattened squamous type
through cuboidal to columnar, the shape, as in mammals, generally
reflecting the activity of the follicle. Under the light microscope a
characteristic of these cells is large apical droplets which are PAS
positive and also stain with iron-haematoxylin. These droplets are
not secretory but as in other higher vertebrate thyroids are formed
by a pinocytotic engulfing of follicle colloid. Secretory droplets are
also present in the cytoplasm but are smaller and formed in the
Golgi bodies.

Electron-micrographs of the teleost thyroid show follicle cells
whose microvilli are fewer than those seen in higher vertebrates
but whose rough surface endoplasmic reticulum is well developed
throughout the cytoplasm as in higher vertebrates. Free ribosomes

are widely distributed in the matrix of the cytoplasm. Droplets either dense or less-dense which appear to be derived from the Golgi elements, are present as are lysosomes, containing small vesicles, membranous structures and wrapped whorled lamellae. The fine structure of the pericapillary region is similar to that of higher vertebrates though endothelial pores have not been seen.

The colloid, whose main component is the glycoprotein, thyroglobulin, stains with many dyes, such as eosin or aniline blue and again as in tetrapods its viscosity appears to alter and this is reflected in its staining properties. The colloid peripheral vacuoles which appear after conventional fixation are regarded, as in mammals, largely as a fixation artefact.

As explained in the previous chapter the teleost pituitary contains and releases a thyrotrophic hormone which appears to regulate thyroid function. The response of the teleost thyroid both to mammalian and teleost TSH can be measured quantitatively either by histological or biochemical parameters and in fact the goldfish thyroid has sufficient responsiveness to form the basis of a bioassay.

The concentration of iodine by the thyroid gland of fish has long been known. In 1910 Marine and Lenhart showed that low-iodine water produced thyroid hyperplasia and goitre and that the condition could be prevented by the addition of iodine to the water, but it was not until 1947 when radioactive iodine became available that iodine and thyroidal hormone kinetics could be studied in detail. An early example of thyroidal iodine metabolism is shown in Figure 2.5. Radioactive thyroid hormones are produced, but much more slowly than in mammals where labelled thyroxine appears well within the first 24 hours after giving tracer iodine. When radioactive iodine is injected into most freshwater teleost fish about 30 per cent of the dose appears in the thyroid at about 24 hours, although there is great variability among species, and some species such as the goldfish and sunfish (*Lepomis gibbosus*) have maximal uptake of labelled iodine by the thyroid gland of only a few per cent. Obviously sea water which contains much more iodine than fresh will result in a relatively much lower maximal uptake of labelled iodine by the thyroid of salt water fish than of fresh water fish. This is particularly well seen in euryhaline fish which take up more iodine in their thyroid when they are in fresh water than when in salt.

The plasma iodide (ionic form) of fresh water teleosts is very

Figure 2.5: Thyroidal Iodine Metabolism of Goldfish after an Injection of [131]I. Note presence of thyroxine only in fish pre-treated with mammalian TSH.

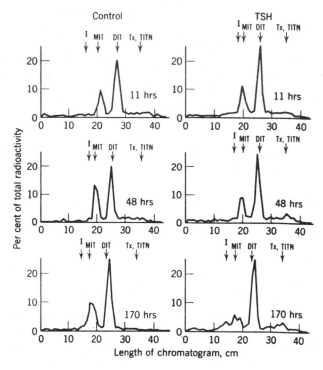

Source: Berg, O. and Gorbman, H. (1954) Normal and altered thyroidal function in domesticated goldfish, *Carassius auratus. Proc. Soc. Exp. Biol. Med., 86,* 156.

variable ranging from 0.5 to over 2,000 µg/100 mg (fresh water iodine 1-2 µg/litre; sea water 45-60 µg/litre). Iodine is also bound to plasma proteins as are the thyroid hormones. The iodine-binding protein of rainbow trout is located on a specific plasma protein electrophoretic peak. Plasma proteins thus contribute to the conservation of plasma iodine required for the synthesis of the thyroid hormones.

   The biochemistry of the incorporation of iodine with tyrosine molecules to result in thyroid hormones appears in fish to follow the pattern shown in all vertebrates. Iodide is trapped by the follicle cells, oxidation of iodide to reactive iodine occurs and then there is iodination of tyrosine creating first 3-monoiodotyrosine (MIT) and next 3,5-diiodotyrosine (DIT). These molecules form thyroxine (T_4) by the coupling of two molecules of DIT with the subsequent loss of an alanine side chain and triiodothyronine (T_3) by the coupling of one molecule of MIT with one of DIT. Again as in mammals there is every reason to suppose in fish that the thyroid hormones (including DIT and MIT) become bound to thyroglobulin at the periphery of the follicle colloid.

Thyroglobulin amino acid composition differs in differing groups of vertebrates. The amino acid analyses of fish thyroglobulins show general similarity in composition to other vertebrates. The teleost thyroglobulins are relatively homogeneous and their amino acid composition is closer to those of mammalian thyroglobulins than lungfish or dogfish. There exists significant differences between the sedimentation coefficients of fish thyroglobulins and thus molecular weights vary. For example, lungfish thyroglobulin has been calculated as having a molecular weight of 860,000 while that of salmonids is 600,000.

The thyroid hormones bound to thyroglobulin are released by proteolytic hydrolysis in the follicle cell and then pass basally into the capillary blood flow. The iodothyronines T_3 and T_4 are, as mentioned above, bound to specific plasma proteins and are transported to various tissues in the body. This thyroidal hormone production can be modified, accelerated, or slowed down by a number of factors. For example, TSH enhances all aspects of thyroid function while dietary iodine, temperature and other hormones all affect this biosynthetic pathway. The plasma T_4 response to TSH is not influenced though by nutritional state, or other non-specific factors such as stress.

The effect of temperature on fish thyroidal activity has long been suspected, particularly because of the well-known dependence of poikilotherm metabolism on temperature. Thyroid cell height in the minnow *Phoxinus phoxinus* increases with temperature as does uptake of ^{131}I by the thyroid of the eel, and the level of thyroid hormone in the plasma of goldfish. However, rainbow trout kept at 18°C have plasma values of T_4 of about 0.9 µg/ 100ml, whereas those kept at 11°C have higher values; approximately 2.5 µg/100ml. The relationship of temperature with thyroid gland activity in fish has yet to be finally established.

Thyroxine levels are lower in starved fish and in fish fed on a low-protein low-calorie diet compared with fish fed on a high-protein high-calorie diet. Starvation or the feeding of a low-protein low-calorie diet seems to depress thyroidal function and also the conversion of thyroxine to triiodothyronine. In mammals T_3 is probably the active hormone at the cellular level and therefore in fish a way of regulating thyroid activity in relation to calorie-protein intake might be to regulate the conversion of T_4 into T_3 at some peripheral site (Figure 2.6).

With regard to the actual plasma levels of thyroxine and triiodothyronine in teleosts these are low, usually below 500 ng/100ml. Two-year-old brook trout for example have T_4 levels about 165 ng/100ml while T_3 levels are somewhere around 180 ng/100ml. Plasma thyroxine is appreciably excreted by the bile and there is very little degradation and recycling of iodide.

Little is known of the binding sites in fish for thyroid hormones, but recently saturable binding of T_3 has been demonstrated in the liver nuclei of rainbow trout using an *in vivo* isotope displacement method. Saturable sites have not been found in mitochondrial, microsomal or cytosol fractions. The sites are intranuclear and are

Figure 2.6: Radiochromatographs Indicating Conversion of T_4 into T_3 in Fed Brook Trout. A, B, fed; C, D, starved.

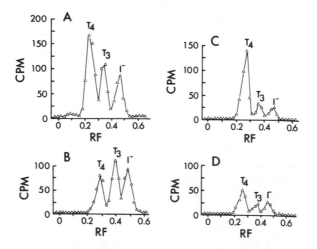

Source: Higgs, D.A. and Eales, J.G. (1977) Influence of food deprivation on radioiodothyronine and radioiodide kinetics in yearling brook trout, *Salvelinus fontinalis* (Mitchill), with a consideration of the extent of L-thyroxine conversion to 3,5,3'-triiodo-L-thyronine. *Gen. Comp. Endocrinol., 32,* 29-40.

a heat-labile protein, probably non-histone, in nature. They have an affinity for T_3 very comparable with that found in mammals. The binding capacity of the sites ranges from 0.4×10^{-12} to 0.6×10^{-12} mol T_3 per gram of liver. About 50 per cent of the sites are normally occupied and approximately tenfold increases in plasma T_3 levels are required to achieve saturation. There is no proof as yet that these sites are in fact the receptors responsible for the initiation of hormone action.

Although, largely due to the work of Eales, teleost thyroid hormone kinetics are well known the same cannot be said of their action at the peripheral cellular level. Mitochondria isolated from trout treated with thyroxine show decreased phosphorylation efficiency and increased specific activity of oxidative enzyme systems. Also if thyroxine is administered *in vitro* to mitochondria a lower concentration of the hormone uncouples oxidation and phosphorylation than is required to bring about this response in mammals.

As mentioned for elasmobranchs the fact that thyroid hormone exerts a calorigenic effect in mammals has prompted many attempts in bony fish to determine whether the thyroid affects respiratory metabolism. Surgical thyroidectomy has been done and oxygen consumption measured over a period of six weeks, drugs and hormones injected and *in vitro* measurement of oxygen consumption of muscle performed. The results of all these experiments have been equivocal but there is no clearly established influence on oxidative metabolism by thyroid hormones in bony fish. In fact if one regards the calorigenic action of thyroid hormones in birds and mammals as being part of the complex of adaptations associated with homeothermy it is not surprising that poikilotherms such as fish should not show this response.

That the thyroid plays a significant role in growth and its associated metabolism in bony fish is well established. Immersion and injection treatment promotes growth in length and weight (Figure 2.7) providing that the dose administered is not too large because, as in mammals, as we shall see, thyroid hormones in fish can act in either an anabolic manner or a catabolic manner. The growth responses do not, however, exclude the fact that the thyroid hormones may be stimulating growth hormone production. Therefore thyroidectomy and hypophysectomy is required to establish beyond reasonable doubt that thyroid hormones are exerting their growth promoting effects directly at the tissue level, such as on muscle and bone. Unfortunately thyroidectomy is impossible to perform in most species of bony fish due to the diffuse nature of the gland. Radiothyroidectomy using ^{131}I and 'chemical thyroidectomy' using goitrogenic drugs such as thiourea have been used as methods of thyroid ablations in young fish. Both these approaches can be criticised because of their possible toxic effects. Nevertheless total radiothyroidectomy both in salmon, trout (Figure 2.8) and platyfish has been shown to retard growth. Reduction in haemopoiesis, reduced calcification, and arrest of sexual development also occurs but it is difficult to establish that these results are directly dependent on thyroid hormone lack and not on radiation damage.

The results of hypophysectomy show that thyroxine or triiodothyronine are in themselves not capable of promoting growth in fish but require the presence of some hypophysial factor such as growth hormone or a pituitary-induced growth promoting factor. Thyroxine cannot restore growth in hypophysectomised guppies; neither has TSH any effect on the growth of hypophysectomised killifish. Thyroid hormones have been shown to change the histological feature of somatotrops thereby suggesting that there is

Figure 2.7: The Influence upon the Growth of Rainbow Trout (*Salmo gairdneri*) of the Addition of Thyroid Powder to the Food. Mean weekly measurements of weight (■) and length (●) of experimental (------) and control (———) groups of fish.

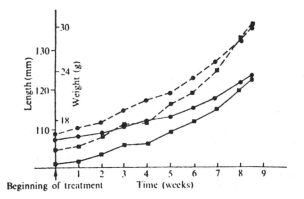

Source: Barrington, E.J.W., Barron, N. and Piggins, D.J. (1961) The influence of thyroid powder and thyroxine upon the growth of rainbow trout (*Salmo gairdneri*). *Gen. Comp. Endocrinol., 1*, 170.

Figure 2.8: Influence of L-thyroxine (T₄) on Growth (Mean Percentage Increase) of Radiothyroidectomised and Untreated Steelhead Trout. Three months after complete thyroid destruction, 10 radiothyroidectomised (69 mm, 3.67 g) and 10 untreated (73 mm, 4.74 g) steelhead trout were immersed in a solution of T₄ (1:10,000,000). Ten radiothyroidectomised (70 mm, 3.62 g) and 10 untreated (76 mm, 5.11 g) trout did not receive T₄ treatment.

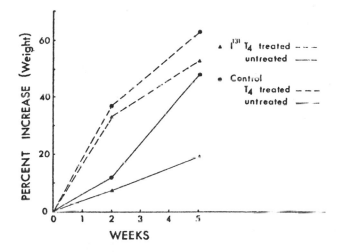

Source: Norris, D.O. (1960) Depression of growth following radiothyroidectomy of larval chinook salmon and steelhead trout. *Trans. Am. Fish Soc., 98*, 104.

stimulation of growth hormone release from these somatotrops.

The growth of muscle, bone and cartilage all seem to be influenced by thyroid hormones. Skull bone growth is decreased following radiothyroidectomy but the inclusion of thyroxine in the diet increases skull dimensions and leads to hyperplasia of connective tissue elements of the interorbital region. Also the treatment of yearling rainbow trout with thyroxine stimulates the uptake of [³⁵S] sulphate into the cells and matrix of branchial skeleton cartilage or bone. Further evidence that thyroid hormone must act in concert with other growth factors is supplied by the fact that *in vitro* experiments on the effects of thyroxine on sulphate binding by trout chondrocytes is negative.

Thyroid hormones, administered at doses that might be considered physiological, enhance protein and RNA synthesis (Figure 2.9).

Figure 2.9: Effect of a Single Injection of Triiodothyronine (T₃) on the Increase in Protein and RNA Content of (a) Liver and (b) Muscle of Starving Tilapia. △, 0.5 µg/g; ■, 1.0 µg/g; □, 2.0 µg/g.

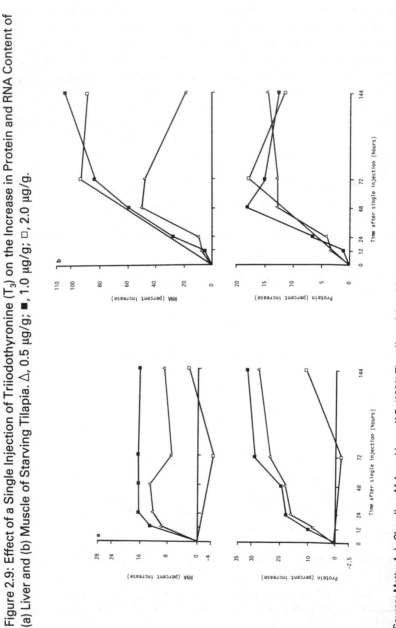

Source: Matty, A.J., Chaudhry, M.A. and Lone, K.P. (1982) The effect of thyroid hormones and temperature on protein and nucleic acid contents of liver and muscle of *Sarotherodon mossambica. Gen. Comp. Endocrinol., 47,* 497-507.

Both trout and goldfish have been shown to incorporate L-[1-14C]-leucine more rapidly into their muscle protein after immersion in thyroxine or triiodothyroxine solutions. Other tissues such as plasma, liver and gills also show increased incorporation of L-leucine. Thyroid hormone also increased the concentration of free amino acids in the plasma. It is possible then that there is increased turnover and/or increased amino acid absorption by the intestine. Deamination may also be increased by thyroid hormones for in goldfish thyroxine increases nitrogen excretion (Figure 2.10). This response may well be temperature and dose dependent.

Although its effect on growth and protein metabolism appears to be one of the best established functions of the thyroid gland there is evidence for some involvement of thyroid hormones in both lipid and carbohydrate metabolism.

Radiothyroidectomy results in increased visceral lipid deposition whereas fish treated with thyroxine have less liver and abdominal fat. It seems then that thyroid hormones stimulate lipid

Figure 2.10: Ammonia Excretion of Goldfish Immersed in Thyroxine Solution at 21°C.

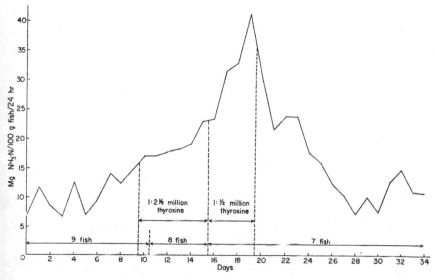

Source: Thornburn, C.C., and Matty, A.J. (1963) The effect of thyroxine on some aspects of nitrogen metabolism in the goldfish (*Carassius auratus*) and the trout (*Salmo trutta*). *Comp. Biochem. Physiol.*, 8, 1-12.

mobilisation in bony fish. The energy supplied by this breakdown of fat could thus spare more protein for growth. Thyroxine treatment also lowers the liver glycogen content and the blood glucose level while increasing heart and muscle glycogen.

Also gluconate oxidation by the liver and cytochrome oxidase activity are increased after thyroid hormone treatments. Again these effects on carbohydrate metabolism may be directed to enable more protein to be used for growth.

Thyroid hormones in bony fish have been shown to be involved also in pigment and guanine deposition, central nervous activity, reproduction, osmoregulation and migration movements. This wide-ranging spectrum of probably physiological changes, suggests either that thyroid hormones in fish play a very basic role themselves in general metabolism or that they activate and modulate a number of different biochemical pathways.

In higher vertebrates the effect of thyroid hormones on the skin and on moulting in reptiles and modification of feather formation in birds is well known. Therefore, it is not surprising that epidermal thickening and changes in pigmentation have been shown to occur in fish after thyroid treatment. The silvering of salmonids increases when subject to thyroid hormones. This is due to increased guanine crystal deposition. [^{14}C]-Glycine is incorporated into skin guanine more rapidly in thyroxine-treated fish than in normal ones. In addition to affecting silvering in salmonids thyroid hormones also cause xanthophore concentration and melanophore dispersion in other species of fish. In all fish that have been examined the hormones result in a thickening of the epidermis. This is in marked contrast to the thinning of the mammalian epidermis seen after thyroid treatment.

In addition to integumentary effects thyroxine also increases the proportion of porphyropsin visual pigment in the retina. Another effect on the eye that has been continually noted is that thyroid hormones are capable of producing esophthalmos in teleosts. This is again in marked contrast to the usual clinical and experimental presumption that exophthalmos is due to an excess of a pituitary substance.

In mammals thyroid hormones sensitise the nervous system and there is a functional impairment of the system in hypothyroid conditions. Similarly in fish a number of behavioural and neurophysiological phenomena have been shown to change with changing thyroid hormone levels.

When salmonids and goldfish are immersed in a thyroxine solution and fed a diet containing thyroxine increased locomotory behaviour ensues as does increased feeding behaviour. Salmon show increased rate, and amount, of swimming but decreased schooling. Also if trout are subject to operant conditioning, i.e. taught, to operate a demand feeding trigger, then triiodothyronine incorporated in the diet results in increased trigger pressing. The behavioural patterns may be a result of the direct effect of thyroid hormone on the brain. If goldfish are injected with thyroxine for ten days and then the electrical potentials evoked in the midbrain after optic stimulation by flashes of light measured, then the hormone appears to change both their form and rate characteristics. The latency of response is reduced, also the time needed to reach maximum response, and there is an increased amplitude of response (Figure 2.11). From these and other results it has been suggested that thyroxine has a facilitating action upon tectal (midbrain) synaptic events.

Thyroid hormones influence the reproductive processes of many vertebrates though there appears to be many species and age

Figure 2.11: Effect of Thyroxine on the Amplitude of the Optically Evoked Potential Recorded at a Depth of 400μm in the Optic Tectum of the Goldfish Brain. ○, Control; ●, thyroxine injected.

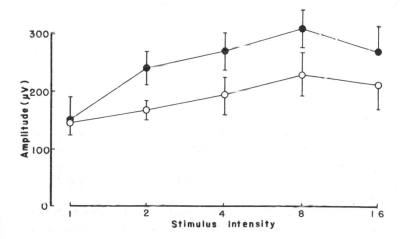

Source: Hara, T.J., Ueda, K. and Gorbman, A. (1965) Influences of thyroxine and sex hormones upon optically evoked potentials in the optic tectum of goldfish. *Gen. Comp. Endocrinol.*, *5*, 313-9.

differences. For example testes functions are more easily impaired in young animals than in adults by thyroid lack. There appears in bony fish also to be a close correlation of thyroid and reproductive activity although cause and effect are often difficult to establish. The making of teleosts hypothyroid either by treatment with goitrogens, radiothyroidectomy or surgical thyroidectomy does not inevitably retard gonad development. Certainly goitrogenic effects may be regarded as toxic manifestations of rapidly dividing tissue. But even here thiouracil has been shown at certain times of the year to have little or no effect on spermatogenesis in the minnow, *Phoxinus phoxinus*. Nevertheless thyroxine clearly stimulates ovarian development in the intact goldfish but has no influence on hypophysectomised regressed adult individuals. The ovarian response to salmon gonadotropin is enhanced by the hormone (Figure 2.12). Thus possibly thyroxine acts synergistically with gonadotropin rather than directly stimulating pituitary function because of the increase of ovarian response to gonadtropin even after pituitary ablation. Furthermore there is some indication that

Figure 2.12: The Effect of Thyroxine (T₄) and Salmon Gonadotropin (SG) on the Ovaries of Hypophysectomised Regressed Goldfish. A, atretic follicle; PV, previtellogenic oocytes; V, vitellogenic oocytes.

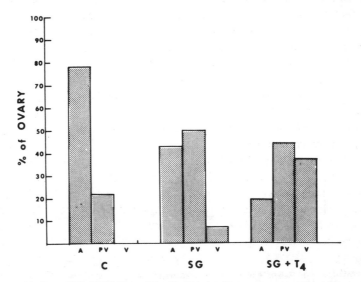

Source: Hurlburt, M.E. (1977) Role of the thyroid gland in ovarian maturation of the goldfish, *Carassius auratus* L. *Can. J. Zool., 55*, 1906-13.

thyroxine may actually inhibit pituitary gonadotroph function. The nature of this synergistic effect is unknown.

If thyroid hormones appear to influence gonadal development particularly in the female then gonadotrophin and gonadal hormones may affect the thyroid. There is much evidence that this is so. Testosterone in some species of fish causes thyroid hyperplasia, increased thyroxine degradation and increased conversion of T_4 into T_3. However, plasma thyroxine values are variable and give little indication here of thyroid function. Androgens could modify thyroid function either by action on the hypothalmus, by altering the peripheral metabolism of the thyroid hormones, by causing anabolic changes which secondarily lead to thyroidal stimulation or by direct stimulation of the thyroid cells. Mammalian pituitary gonadotropins, FSH and LH have been shown to stimulate fish thyroid activity and plasma T_4 values. In one instance salmon gonadotropin has been shown to increase thyroid activity in gonadectomised Pacific salmon, *Oncorhynchus nerka*. Cortisol injections have also been shown to increase plasma T_4 concentrations. Growth hormone as previously mentioned also has a thyrotrophic effect. Thus it would seem that some, if not much, of the correlation seen between reproductive activity and thyroid activity in fish may well come from elevated pituitary hormones in the plasma directly affecting thyroid metabolism. It is possibly this effect of gonadotropin that results in the marked difference in the weight of female thyroids compared with that of adult male thyroids of the parrot fish, *Scarus guacamaia* (Figure 2.13). This difference is not seen in immature fish.

In addition to changes with the reproductive condition seasonal fluctuations in thyroid activity have been observed in fish and correlated with hibernation, migration and changes in the external environment. Again this is a situation similar to that seen in higher groups of vertebrates.

The first seasonal measurements in teleost thyroids were made by measuring thyroid epithelial heights of the minnow and the cod. Many other species also show seasonal changes of thyroid histology. However, this is not as true a reflection, as previously pointed out, of thyroid activity as the measure of plasma and thyroid gland hormones, nevertheless it is interesting here to note that seasonal variation seems to occur in both immature and mature cod thus tending to negate any relationship with reproduction. Seasonal thyroid hormone levels have been measured in salmonids. In the

Figure 2.13: Dry Weights of Thyroids in Male and Female *Scarus guacamaia.*

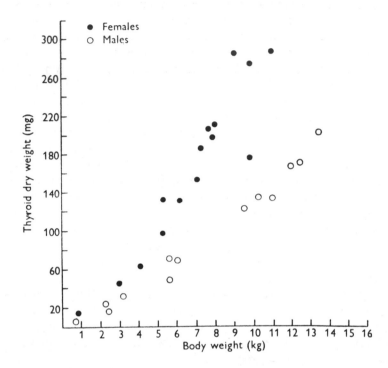

Source: Matty, A.J. (1957) Thyroidectomy and its effect upon oxygen consumption of a teleost fish, *Pseudoscarus guacamaia. J. Endocrinol., 15,* 1.

trout, *Salmo gairdneri,* there appear to be two peaks in plasma concentration (Figure 2.14), while in Lake Ontario coho salmon there is but one peak of serum T_4 and T_3. Concentrations of T_4 and T_3 rise during the autumn in rainbow trout reaching a maximum in November. This rise is unrelated functionally to gonad maturation as it occurs in males and females and in immature and mature fish. During this period there is an increase in the T_4/T_3 ratio indicating a decrease in liver degradation of T_4 or possibly less peripheral utilisation. In the spring the hormone levels again rise but the T_4/T_3 ratio remains unchanged. It is difficult to relate these undoubted seasonal variations to a physiological role of the thyroid particularly when the T_4/T_3 ratio also changes seasonally. It has been suggested that two thyroid cycles occur in teleost fish, one concerned with temperature compensating mechanisms and the other with reproduction. Plasma T_4 has been found to be inversely related to temperature in the rainbow trout.

Light and photoperiod may also affect the seasonal level of thyroid hormones for it has been shown that teleost fish exhibit diel variations in circulating levels of T_4 and T_3. Peak values vary, however, the goldfish peak being at about 1600 hours and that of rainbow trout at 2000 hours. It has been hypothesised for mammals that circadian variation in circulating thyroid hormones may be caused by diel feed-fast regimes. But there is no evidence as yet in fish that this is so (Figure 2.15). In fact little is known about this rhythm. Perhaps it is related to the known daily rhythms of cortisol and prolactin in fishes or in some way with thermo-regulation. In this latter case diel variation in temperature tole-rance has been demonstrated in fishes and thyroid hormones may adjust to give maximum growth stimulation at optimum tempera-ture levels.

Figure 2.14: Annual Variation in Plasma Thyroid Hormone Levels of Rainbow Trout.

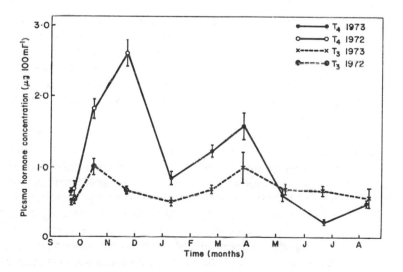

Source: Osborn, R.H., Simpson, T.H. and Youngson, A.F. (1978) Seasonal and diurnal rhythms of thyroidal status in the rainbow trout, *Salmo gairdneri* Richardson. *J. Fish Biol.*, *12*, 531-40.

Figure 2.15: Diel Changes in Plasma T_4 and T_3 Levels of Fed or
Starved Rainbow Trout Held at 11°C on a 12L:12D Photoperiod.
Fed trout were presented with food at 0930 h. Geometric means
(±95% confidence intervals) are shown for groups of 9 or 10 trout.
At each sampling point significant differences (t test) between
mean values of starved and fed trout are indicated by probability
values in the lower panel (NS = nonsignificant difference,
$P > 0.05$). Analysis of variance indicated no significant difference
between sampling times for either plasma T_4 or plasma T_3 of
starved trout. However, plasma T_4 ($P > 0.01$) and plasma T_3
($P = 0.05$) did differ between sampling times for fed trout.

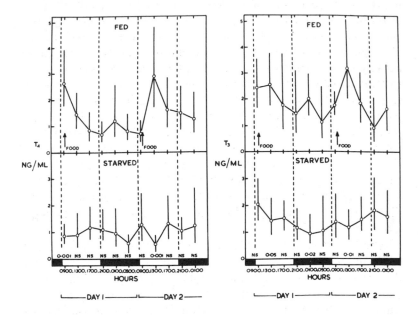

Source: Eales, J.G., Hughes, M. and Vin, L. (1981) Effect of food intake on diel variation
in plasma thyroid hormone levels in rainbow trout, *Salmo gairdneri. Gen. Comp.
Endocrinol.*, 45, 167-74.

In addition to the correlation of seasonal variation of the
activity of the thyroid gland with reproduction and feeding there
exists without doubt changes in thyroid activity with migratory
changes, with salinity changes in the environment, and with the
modification process that occurs in salmonids just prior to their

seaward migration. The part played by thyroxine and triiodo-thyronine in these phenomena will be discussed in Chapter 8 but a few features of the effect of thyroid hormone on mineral metabolism and ion balance may now be mentioned. As with so many aspects of thyroid physiology in fish the results are equivocal. Plasma Na^+ and Cl^- levels are transiently lowered in TSH-injected sea water-adapted rainbow trout and in fresh water-adapted fish there is a slight indication of a fall in Na^+ levels. Also in several species of the teleost, *Xiphophorus*, following hypophysectomy their ability to survive in fresh water is abolished and they must be kept in one-third sea water. However, TSH injection of these hypophysectomised fish does not enable them to survive in fresh water (unlike prolactin). Some enzymes, however, that are associated with sodium flux or which are activated by sodium are changed by thyroxine treatment in fish. Gill acetylcholinesterase activity is significantly increased in channel catfish after thyroxine treatment. Also there is a correlation between thyroid activity and sodium-potassium activated adenosine triphosphatase in salmonids. This latter important osmoregulatory involved enzyme is probably more concerned with altering flux rates of plasma Na^+/Cl^- ions rather than concentrations. As we shall see in Chapter 8 although thyroid hormones are involved in migration and smoltification of salmonids and although ambient salinity may have some indirect effect on thyroid activity there is no good evidence of a direct involvement of thyroid hormone with ionic or osmotic regulation in bony fish.

The β-adrenoceptor inhibitor propranolol, cholecalciferol, and organochlorides have all recently been found to alter serum thyroxine levels thus making any unitary explanation of the role of fish thyroid hormones further distant. Perhaps the only adequate summary of the function of this gland has been expressed by one researcher in the field as 'the real significance of the thyroid in fish lies in its ability to aid adaptation of the organism to environmental vicissitudes such as osmotic and temperature stress and periods of rapid internal change (growth) and sexual maturation'.

The Ultimobranchial Gland

Just as the thyroid gland develops as a ventral outgrowth of the pharynx at the level of the first and second branchial pouches so another structure, the ultimobranchial gland, is derived from the last branchial pouch area in embryonic fish. This tissue migrates backwards, during the course of development of the fish, to a position lying over the pericardium. Sometimes the outgrowth from the pharynx is paired, sometimes, as in the elasmobranchs, it develops from one side of the embryonic pharynx only. Although we have spoken of fish, we should more correctly refer to gnathostomes for in the Agnatha, the cyclostomes and myxinoids no outgrowths of the pharynx comparable to ultimobranchial tissue has been identified.

It is only within recent years that the hormone content and the function of this gland have been identified in fishes. The gland in mammals has a calcium-regulating function and produces a hormone known as calcitonin which is produced by the parafollicular or 'C' cells which form part of the thyroid gland. The first indication in fish that the gland was also involved in calcium metabolism was when the Mexican cave fish, *Astyanax mexicanus*, was kept in total darkness for two years and hyperplasia of the ultimobranchial gland, along with gross body skeletal deformities were observed. However, it was in elasmobranchs and chimaeroids that this gland was first described a hundred years ago when they were referred to as 'suprapericardial bodies' due to their location on and above the pericardium. There is variation in the positioning of the gland. In the dogfish, *Squalus acanthias*, the gland is found on the left side only between the pericardium and the ventral surface of the pharynx just anterior to its junction with the oesophagus. In another dogfish, *Scyliorhinus canicula*, however, the gland is situated ventral to the pharynx medial to the fifth gill arch; in some specimens of this species the gland is a bilateral structure, while in other specimens the gland is visible only on the left side of the pharynx.

Microscopically the gland consists of many follicles containing granular material in their cavities while the surrounding epithelial cells are columnar. There are two cell types, one mitochondrial rich, the other mitochondrial poor. The holocephalian gland is bilateral and also has cells of two different types.

In teleosts the gland is again either bilateral or single lying in the midline and is generally located in the transverse septum between the abdominal cavity and the sinus venosus just ventral to the oesophagus. In the rainbow trout the gland is located between the oesophagus and the sinus venosus immediately rostral to the transverse septum. The gland in this species is, however, often solid, containing no obvious follicles, and is composed of secreting cells and non-granular irregularly shaped cells which are possibly supporting in nature.

The hormone calcitonin was first shown to be a potent hypocalcaemic factor in mammals and shortly after demonstrating its presence and biological action of inhibiting bone resorption the hormone was prepared in a chemically pure form. It was shown to be a straight chain peptide with 32 amino acid residues and a molecular weight of approximately 3,400. Almost immediately after these discoveries in the late 1960s, salmon calcitonin was isolated and its structure determined. It was shown to have the same number of amino acids as porcine calcitonin but there are a number of amino acid substitutions (Figure 2.16).

All fish appear to contain calcitonin in their ultimobranchial glands often in much higher concentration than that found in mammals. If the hormone had an action in fish similar to that in

Figure 2.16: (a) Structure of Salmon Calcitonin; (b) Structure of Porcine Calcitonin (Changed Amino Acids Underlined).

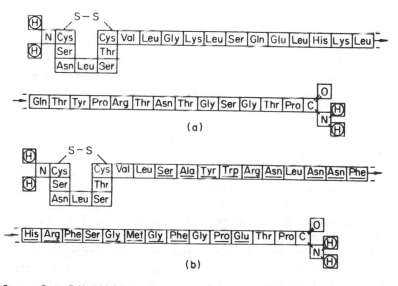

Source: Copp, D.H. (1969) The ultimobranchial glands and calcium regulation, in W.S. Hoar and D..l Randall (eds.) *Fish Physiology*, vol. II. Academic Press, New York, pp. 377-98.

mammals then this would seem a paradox as the chondrichthyes contain no true bone and the bone of teleosts is acellular. Indeed when extracts of ultimobranchial glands or mammalian or fish calcitonin were administered to fish then there was no lowering of serum calcium levels. This does preclude the view that calcitonin in fish may facilitate in some way calcium transport mechanisms and so take a part in calcium regulation in fish. This is indicated by the fact that if calcitonin is administered to salt water eels then no hypocalcaemia is elicited but if the hormone is presented to fresh water-adapted eels then hypocalcaemia results. Prolonged injections of synthetic salmon calcitonin do not have any noticeable influence on total plasma calcium in seawater-adapted sticklebacks an effect, or rather lack of effect, which has been confirmed by many other attempts to influence plasma calcium by calcitonin. In some experiments changes in plasma chloride have been observed which has prompted some investigators to suggest that calcitonin in fish is primarily concerned with hydromineral metabolism in general. There is little evidence that this is so.

Salmon gills when perfused *in vivo* with calcitonin show a decreased influx of calcium and phosphate and increased outflux. Also calcitonin has been shown to increase clearance of calcium by the kidney. Thus the absence of a hypocalcaemic action of the hormone may be due to experimental design or other factors. It is possible then in fish that the hypocalcaemic action of the gland and its hormone may be obscured by changes in the release of endogenous calcitonin or by the release of hypercalcaemic factors from other glands in the fish. There has, as has been already mentioned, growing evidence that in teleosts prolactin is involved in the endocrine control of calcium metabolism. Prolactin has a hypercalcaemic activity in a number of species. The corpuscles of Stannius produce a hypocalcaemic factor. Taking all these factors into account it may be that the establishment of a hypocalcaemic condition by increased renal output and decreased gill input is the primary physiological function of this hormone in fish similar to that seen in mammals.

Calcitonin may also be connected to migration and reproductive behaviour. Although high levels of calcitonin are found in salmon blood they are higher in females than in males. Also plasma calcium decreases progressively throughout male salmon migration. In the female although there is a marked increase in calcitonin levels up to the time of spawning when this occurs there is a rapid fall in plasma calcitonin (Figure 2.17). This suggests that calcitonin may play an important role in the reproductive cycle of fish conserving and mobilising calcium particularly for egg formation. Histological changes of the ultimobranchial gland, particularly in the height of the epithelial cells and their granulation, can be correlated with reproductive changes in the Japanese salmon, *Oncorhynchus masou.* Degeneration of the epithelial cells occurs in this fish during ovulation. Mature goldfish also show a more active ultimobranchial gland, as judged by histological criteria, than the gland of young fish. A relationship appears undoubtedly to exist between the ultimobranchial gland and gonadal activity but it is far from clear what causal factors exist between these two organs.

Figure 2.17: Changes in Plasma Calcitonin and Calcium during Migration of the Salmon, *Oncorhynchus nerka.* ●, females; ○, males.

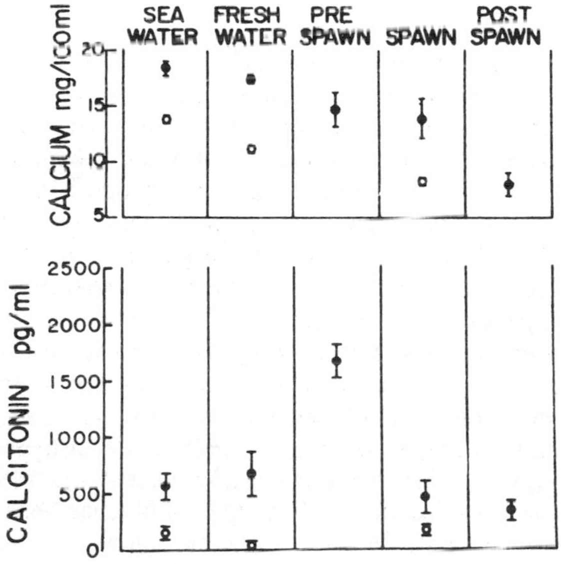

Source: Watts, E.G., Copp, D.H. and Deftos, L.J. (1975) Changes in plasma calcitonin and calcium during migration of salmon. *Endocrinol., 96*, 214-18.

3 PANCREATIC AND GASTROINTESTINAL HORMONES

The Pancreas

Although the vertebrate pancreas must be regarded as part of the alimentary tract the endocrine pancreas is concerned with functions other than with the process of digestion. The pancreatic enzymes and the gastrointestinal hormones perform functions quite different in the higher vertebrates from those of the endocrine pancreas, whose hormones are concerned with metabolism and growth. All cyclostomes and fishes have an endocrine pancreas of some sort although its anatomy, histology and physiology varies considerably within the group. The hormone insulin is present throughout but glucagon is confined to the fishes proper.

Cyclostomes

The endocrine pancreatic tissue of the myxinoids is found as follicles surrounding the point at which the bile duct joins the intestinal tract whereas in the adult petromyzont cyclostomes the tissue is located dorsally and ventrally to the intestinal tract at the point of transition from fore-gut to hind-gut (Figure 3.1). The ventral portion of the pancreas in lampreys also extends into the liver, while the dorsal portion often surrounds a small blind caecum of the intestine forming a whitish swelling and is often referred to as the cranial pancreas.

The follicles of the myxinoid cyclostomes contain cells very largely of one type. These cells show almost all the characteristics of the mammalian insulin-producing B cell. The cytoplasm shows a distinct metachromasia with paraldehyde fuchsin staining, is pseudoisocyanin positive and stains blue in Victoria blue. A specific antiserum against insulin from the hagfish has been prepared and immunofluorescence microscopy has shown that this serum reacted with hagfish islet cells. Scattered among the B cells are cells which stain weakly and are less granular than the majority of the cells. A rare second granular cell is also present with spherical granules contrasting with the ellipsoid granules of the B cells. The nature of this cell is unknown.

Figure 3.1: Fish Pancreas Types. (a) Bony fish, tetrapod type. (b) Bony fish, Brockmann body type. (c) Lamprey. (d) Hagfish. (e) Shark. I, islet tissue; L, liver; EP, exocrine pancreas; G, gall bladder; B, bile duct; IT, intestine.

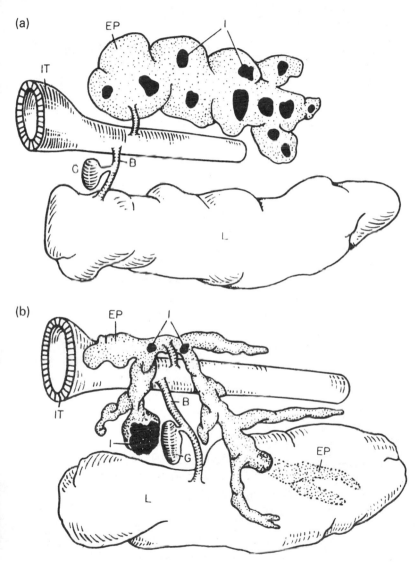

Figure 3.1 continued

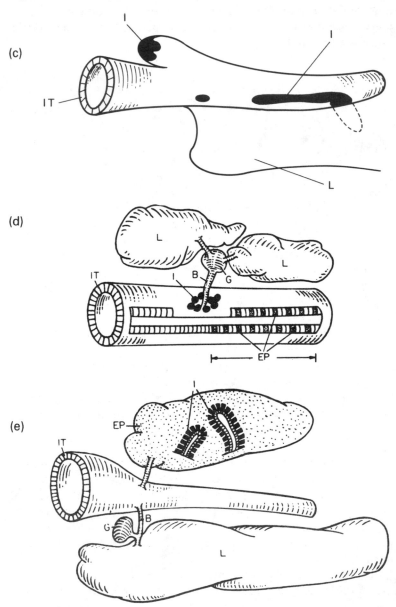

Source: All except (c) from Epple, A. (1969) in W.S. Hoare and D.J. Randall (eds.), *Fish Physiology*. Academic Press, London and New York, p. 275.

Although the larval lamprey pancreas has cells which are arranged as follicles this arrangement is lost in the adult. There is one type of cell which gives a typical B cell reaction and these cells contain electron-dense granules with a diameter of about 170 nm which corresponds well to the mammalian B granules. No A cells are present.

Although it is now well established that insulin is produced by the B cells of cyclostomes and while the amino acid sequence of hagfish has been determined the role of this hormone in the normal physiology of cyclostomes is far from certain. Hagfish (*Myxine glutinosa*) insulin contains 52 amino acids, 21 in the A chain and 31 in the B chain. Eighteen of the residues are different from those found in mammalian insulin. Although this primitive insulin has a similar monomeric structure to that of pig insulin it does not form hexamers. It has only about 10 per cent of the potency of pig insulin in stimulating glucose oxidation and deoxy-glucose transport in rat fat-cells.

Pharmacological experimentation, however, does show a relationship between the cyclostome endocrine pancreas and blood sugar levels. Many years ago Barrington injected a glucose load into larval lampreys and caused a vacuolation or breakdown of the B cells. Alloxan a drug which has a marked toxic effect on mammalian B cells also sometimes causes necrosis of B cells in lampreys and elevation of blood sugar. Also injection of mammalian insulin can cause an *increase* in blood sugar (Figure 3.2). This is most unusual compared with the action of insulin in mammals where blood glucose is reduced. However, most workers have demonstrated hypoglycaemic effects either using mammalian insulin or cyclostome pancreas extracts. There are also indications that the regulation of the amino acid metabolism may be a function of insulin in cyclostomes (Figure 3.3). Although no A cells are present in the cyclostome pancreas this does not preclude glucagon being produced elsewhere in the body. This though is unlikely for efforts to produce physiological (or pharmacological) effects by injection of mammalian glucagon into cyclostomes have been unsuccessful.

The insulin content in the blood of the river lamprey *Lampetra fluviatilis* varies with the season. How this is related to spawning, carbohydrate metabolism or protein metabolism is unknown.

Figure 3.2: The Anomalous Effect of Insulin on Adult River Lamprey, Resulting in Hyperglycaemia after the Injection of Mammalian Insulin Intraperitoneally. This is most likely an indication of gluconeogenesis resulting from catecholamine release by stress.

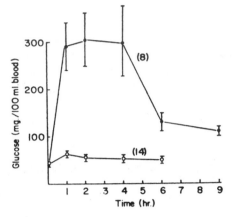

Source: Bentley, P.J. and Follett, B.K. (1965) The effects of hormones on the carbohydrate metabolism of the lamprey, *Lampetra fluviatilis. J. Endocrinol., 31,* 127.

Chondrichthyes

The elasmobranch endocrine pancreas may either be groups of cells forming islets embedded in a compact exocrine pancreas as in mammals or may take the form of an outer layer of small ducts in the pancreas. The arrangement of the endocrine tissue around a duct resembles the early stages of human islet formation (Figure 3.1).

Cytologically three types of endocrine pancreas cell can be recognised, A, B and D. Agranular cells and amphiphils are also seen in the pancreas but their function is problematic. A cells which are azocarmine stain positive and argyrophilic but which do not stain either with pseudoisocyanin or aldehyde fuchsin are known in mammals to be the source of the hormone glucagon. In the chondrichthyes endocrine pancreas a similarly staining cell occurs but as yet glucagon has not been demonstrated in these cells by an immunocytochemical technique. B cells which stain with aldehyde fuchsin and pseudoisocyanin but which are not argyrophilic are the source of insulin in higher vertebrates and are present in the endocrine pancreas of chondrichthyes as indeed they

Figure 3.3: Effect of Bovine Insulin (0.5 IU/kg) on Plasma Glucose and Amino Nitrogen of Hagfish, *Eptatretus stouti.* Controls = open circles; treated = closed circles.

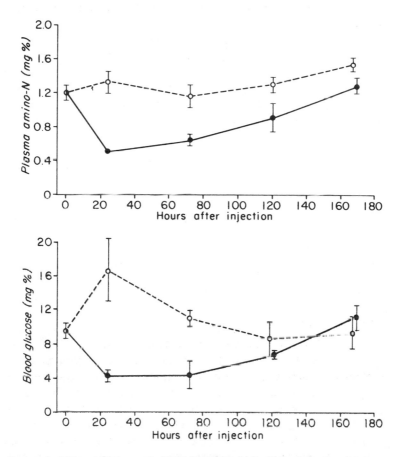

Source: Inui, Y. and Gorbman, A. (1977) Sensitivity of Pacific hagfish, *Eptatretus stouti,* to mammalian insulin. *Gen. Comp. Endocrinol., 33,* 423-7.

are in all vertebrates. Finally, in this group of fish, cells similar in staining properties to the D cells of mammals have been identified. These D cells are argyrophilic, metachromatic with toluidine blue, and only positive to pseudoisocyanin after acid hydrolysis. Very few of them occur in some elasmobranchs such as rays and *Torpedo* while none at all appear to be present in *Scyliorhinus.*

The pancreas of the holocephalii is compact, contains many islets with A, B, and D cells but also contains a peculiar cell type known as the X cell. These X cells have not been shown to occur in other vertebrates and they make up about 50 per cent of all the islet cells in holocephalians. These cells which are filled with fine granules are argyrophilic and stain reddish-brown with Azan. These cells are seen both in *Hydrolagus colliei* and *Chimera monstrosa*.

Whereas the pancreas of the hagfish has been studied in detail, its insulin isolated, crystallised and its amino acid sequence determined, the biology, biochemistry and chemistry of the elasmobranch endocrine pancreas has received little attention. However, as early as 1922 Macleod demonstrated that an acid-ethanol extract of dogfish pancreas contained a substance capable of causing hypoglycaemia in rabbits.

The blood glucose values of elasmobranchs vary widely not only between species but also within a species. For example the blood glucose values of *Scyliorhinus canicula* range between a few milligrams to over 100 mg/100 ml. This makes it difficult to make comparisons and draw evidence from experimental studies. This variability does not seem to be a seasonal fluctuation unlike the situation in cyclostomes and some teleosts. Nutritional states do however, influence blood glucose values in elasmobranchs. Unlike the situation in myxinoid cyclostomes, where blood glucose values fall in fasting animals, starving elasmobranchs maintain their blood sugar values for several weeks and in *Squalus acanthias* when maintained in an unfed state for a month there is even a significant increase in blood sugar at the end of the period. Clearly gluconeogenesis occurs (Figure 3.4). In general insulin regardless of its source and mode of administration produces significant hypoglycaemia in elasmobranchs (Table 3.1). The effect is most evident at about 24 hours after treatment. Nothing is clearly known about the effect of insulin on muscle or liver glycogen levels.

Mammalian glucagon produces a transient hyperglycaemia in dogfish when high doses are given. This experiment has not been carried out with chondrichthyean glucagon for this hormone has yet to be isolated from this group of fish.

The holocephalian, *Hydrolagus colliei*, exhibits hypoglycaemia in response to insulin and a rapid transient hyperglycaemia in response to glucagon.

Surgical removal of the pancreas and removal of the pituitary

Figure 3.4: The Effect of Starvation on Blood Glucose of Various Species of Fish _ _ _ _ *Eptatretus stouti*; __ __ ._ *Squalus acanthias*; _._._. *Raia erinacea*; _____ *Anguilla anguilla*.

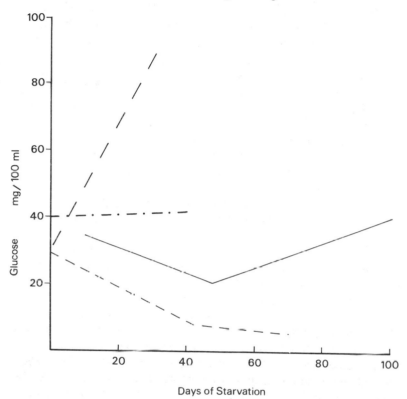

(in order to investigate the presence of a diabetogenic factor) has produced confusing results. Early experiments of pancreatectomy carried out without anaesthetic resulted in marked hyperglycaemia of *Mustelus canis* but further work on *Raia erinacea* showed no hyperglycaemia over a long-term period.

Dunn and his co-workers in 1943 observed that the drug alloxan selectively destroyed the pancreatic B cells of the rabbit. Since this time this cytotoxic substance has been used to induce experimental diabetes or to help in the histological identification of the B cells. Alloxan has been used in several attempts to destroy the islet B cells in a number of elasmobranchs but results have

Table 3.1: Effect of Insulin on Chondrichthyean Blood Sugar Levels

Species	Insulin and dose	Route[1]	Blood glucose	Method	Author
T. pastinaca	Bovine, 2-200 U/kg	i.p.	↓	Hagedorn-Jensen	Liebson *et al.* (1963)
R. erinacea	Bovine, 5 U/kg	i.m.	↓		Grant *et al.* (1969)
S. acanthias	Bovine, 5 U/kg	i.a.	↓	Glucose oxidase	Patent (1970)
	Dogfish, 0.3 U/kg	i.a.	↓		
	Ratfish, 2 U/kg	i.a.	↓		
H. colliei	Bovine, 5 U/kg	i.a.	↓		
	Ratfish, 2 U/kg	i.a.	↓		
	Dogfish, 0.3 U/kg	i.a.	↓		

[1]i.p. — intraperitoneally; i.m. — intramuscularly; i.a. — intra-aortally.

Source: Patent, (1973) *Amer. Zool., 13,* 639

been inconclusive. There is no consistent change in blood glucose or in B cell destruction after treatment with this drug.

The only thing that is known with certainty about the chondrichthyean endocrine pancreas is that the islet tissue consists of a number of cell types one of which produces 'insulin' which when injected reduces blood sugar levels.

Bioassay using the mouse hemi-diaphragm assay shows dogfish and shark insulins to have a much lower (one-twentieth) potency compared with ox insulin. As large amounts of both ox and cod insulin antisera are required to neutralise the effect of dogfish insulin on mouse hemi-diaphragm it suggests that these insulins do not have many antigenic sites in common. Thus the form and the function of the chondrichthyean insulin may be quite different from that of the higher vertebrates. There may be some regulation of carbohydrate metabolism but why is there such wide variation in blood glucose? Is glucose a primary energy source? Does insulin affect protein, urea or lipid metabolism?

Somatostatin has been detected by radioimmunoassay in the pancreas tissue of the dogfish *Squalus acanthias* but nothing is known of its physiology.

Actinopterygii

The pancreas of this group of fish can take one of three forms, it can be compact, lobulated so that it spreads out into various parts of the body cavity or it can be scattered in small portions over the whole body cavity (Figure 3.1). The pancreas histology, of teleosts in particular, has been examined at frequent intervals for nearly 150 years. In 1846 Brockmann described bodies in teleosts which contain largely but not exclusively islet tissue. Exocrine tissue may occur within these bodies; thus the term 'principle islet' which is sometimes used to describe these tissue masses is misleading. These Brockmann bodies are derivatives of the dorsal epithelium of the embryonic gut and correspond to the splenic portion of the avian and reptilian pancreas. As these bodies contain largely endocrine tissue they have been isolated and examined biochemically and physiologically. *Cottus scorpius* and *Lophius piscatorius* are two species of fish which have large and well-defined Brockmann bodies. It has been possible to 'isletectomise' these fish.

The histology of the teleost islet is similar to that of the elasmobranchs with A, B and D cells present. The B cell stains after oxidation with aldehyde fuchsin. Also when stained with pseudo-isocyanin after oxidation the B cell shows metachromasia. The cells are neither acidophilic nor are they argyrophilic. The A cells contain acidophilic granules which stain with acid haemotoxylin and with silver stains. They do not stain with aldehyde fuchsin or pseudoisocyanin. Finally the D cells (sometimes called A_1 cells) stain metachromatically with toluidine blue but do not stain with pseudoisocyanin after oxidation.

As seen with pituitary adenohypophysial cytology the most specific method for cellular identification at the present time is by the use of immunological staining techniques in which fluorescent dye labelled antibodies specifically react with the hormone polypeptide in the cell. In teleosts using this method of immunohistochemical demonstration insulin has been located in the B cells and glucagon in the A cells of, for example, *Xiphophorus, Callionymus* and *Pleuronectes*. This technique can be criticised in that it uses antimammalian hormone sera. In addition to A, B and D cells two other types of amphiphilic cells have been described as occurring in the teleost pancreas but their function is unknown. Also the function of the D (A_1) cell in teleost fish or for all fish for that matter, is not clear, although it is quite likely that a third pancreatic hormone is secreted by this cell type. Some authors have suggested that the D cell produces a gastrin-like peptide analogous to the D cells of the mammalian islets of Langerhans. Other authors have suggested that they produce somatostatin (the release-inhibiting factor for growth hormone) as has been demonstrated with immunofluorescent techniques for mammalian D cells.

This suggestion has received confirmation in that using a mammalian antibody to synthetic somatostatin cells containing somatostatin have been demonstrated in the pancreas of a number of teleost species and in the case of *Xiphophorus helleri* these cells have been shown to be identical to D cells.

Ultrastructural examination of the teleost endocrine pancreas shows cells with characteristic granules. The B cell granules show a marked variation from species to species and are more or less crystalloid in nature. It has been suggested that these variations in B granules might be due to differences in the macromolecular arrangement of the insulin or in the type of binding protein. In *Xiphophorus* although most of the B granules are circular or oval in shape a few are rod shaped while the A granules are often hexagonal in shape (Figure 3.5). The granules of the D cells are much smaller than the other islet cell granules. There is much morphological evidence supporting the view that granule formation in islet cells occurs in the Golgi apparatus.

Electronmicroscope studies of the pancreas of a number of teleosts have demonstrated a heavy nervous innervation of the islets suggesting the presence of direct nervous control.

The effect of alloxan on the teleost B cell has been variable. A

Figure 3.5: Electron Micrographs of A and B Cells of the Pancreatic Islets of *Xiphophorus helleri.* (a) B cell with rod-shaped cores. (b) A cell with hexagonal secreting granules.

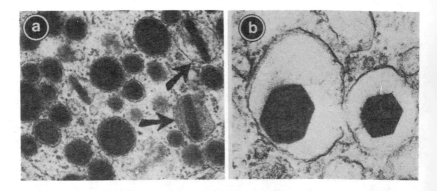

Source: Klein, C. and Lange, R.H. (1977) Principal cell types in the pancreatic islet of a teleost fish, *Xiphophorus helleri* H. *Cell Tiss. Res., 176,* 529-51.

10 per cent aqueous solution (400 mg/kg) produced hyper-glycaemia in 92 per cent of the catfish *Ictalurus nebulosus* injected and degranulation of the B cells was apparent twelve hours after the injection (Figure 3.6). Degeneration of the cells became more severe over a period of 96 hours. Although alloxan is also a B cell cytotoxic agent in goldfish, trout and the guppy, other fish includ-ing *Opsanus, Scorpaena,* carp and tench are alloxan resistant. Streptozotocin, an antibiotic which also has been shown to be a cytotoxin of mammalian B cells, appears to modify the B cell fine structure of the cod. The drug appears to inhibit granule release and to interfere with normal secretory granule production.

Certain cobalt salts when administered to experimental animals have the ability to produce fluctuations in blood glucose levels and histological alterations in the pancreatic islets. Some teleost fish islets concentrate cobalt but degranulation of both the A and the B cells occurs after the administration of these salts. Also, as in

Figure 3.6: Effect of Alloxan on Catfish Blood Glucose. Broken lines beyond 120 hours indicate reduction of number of fish sampled at each period.

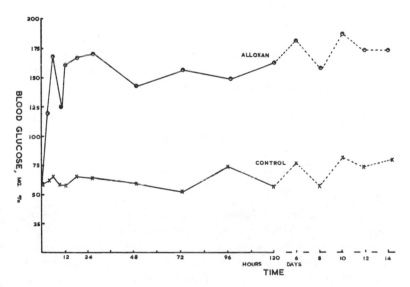

Source: Murrell, L.R. and Nace, P.F. (1959) Experimental Diabetes in the Catfish: normal and alloxan-diabetic blood glucose and pancreatic histology. *Endocrinol., 64,* 542-50.

mammals, heavy doses of glucose appear to result in hyperfunction and consequent exhaustion of the B cells while heavy doses of mammalian glucagon may be cytotoxic to fish A cells.

A number of teleost fish insulins have been isolated, crystallised and their amino acid sequences determined. The amino acid sequence for cod is seen in Figure 3.7. A feature of teleost insulin is that there is an extra residue at the beginning of the B chain. The residues vary, methionine in cod and toad-fish and valine in the angler fish, *Lophius piscatorius*. Another feature of teleost insulin is that residue 30 is missing. Substitution may occur at several residues. As Barrington has remarked, however, mention of these substitutions must not be allowed to obscure the strong conservative element in the evolution of the insulin molecule and it is remarkable that of the 21 invariant residues in the molecules of all vertebrates studied no less than 20 are also invariant in *Myxine glutinosa*.

The biosynthetic pathway for insulin in the Brockmann bodies of teleosts has been studied and insulin precursors identified. Proinsulin has been identified. The effect of tolbutamide, a drug which stimulates insulin production in mammals, does not increase the incorporation of [^{14}C] glucose and [^{3}H] leucine into the insulin fraction of *Lophius* islets.

Two fish glucagons have been isolated and characterised. Angler fish glucagon has 29 residues, like porcine glucagon, but differs from the latter in its composition. It has the same *N*-terminal histidine as porcine glucagon, but a lysine residue instead of threonine as *C*-terminus. The glucagon of the spiny dogfish (*Squalus acanthias*) also has 29 residues but appears to differ from porcine glucagon less than does angler fish glucagon.

Pancreatic Physiology

Insulin and Glucagon

The role of insulin in fishes and in all vertebrates will be more clearly understood when accurate measurements are made of the circulating levels of the hormones under various developmental, nutritional and environmental conditions. Some progress has been made by making direct measurements of endogenous insulin in teleost fish by radioimmunoassay. An obstacle to progress has been the fact that the readily available radioimmunoassay components have generally proved of little or no use in fish insulin

Figure 3.7: Comparison of Amino Acid Sequences of the A and B Chains of Cod and Ox Insulin. The sequences of the ox chains are identical with that of cod except in the positions indicated.

A chain

Cod Gly·Ile·Val·Asp·Gln·Cys·Cys·His·Arg·Pro·Cys·Asp·Ile·Phe·Asp·Leu·Gln·Asn·Tyr·Cys·Asn

Ox   ——Glu—— Ala·Ser·Val ——Ser·Leu·Tyr·Gln—— Glu——
           4   8 9 10   12 13 14 15   17

B chain

Cod Met·Ala·Pro·Pro·Gln·His·Leu·Cys·Gly·Ser·His·Leu·Val·Asp·Ala·Leu·Tyr·Leu·Val·Cys Gly·Asp·Arg·Gly·Phe·Phe·Tyr·Asn·Pro·Lys

Ox   Phe·Val·Asn——————Glu——————————Glu——————Thr——————Ala
      1   2   3   13   21   27   30

Source: Reid, K.B.M., Grant, P.T. and Youngson, A. (1968) The sequence of amino acids in insulin isolated from islet tissue of the cod (*Gadus callarias*). *Biochem. J., 110*, 289-96.

studies because of weak cross-reactivities between many fish insulins and antibodies to mammalian insulins. Some workers have shown that it is possible to produce an antiserum to mammalian insulin (an antibovine-porcine mixture) which cross reacts for certain fish insulins such as the scorpion fish and trout, enabling the fish hormone to be assayed. However, homologous radio-immunoassays have been developed using pure cod insulin or crystalline scorpion fish insulin. These homologous assays have been used to determine the insulin content of a number of teleost plasmas (Table 3.2).

If cod are starved for a period of four days then their plasma insulin values drop by about a half although their plasma glucose values only fall by a few per cent. The fall in plasma amino acid nitrogen is much greater. Also feeding trout with a high protein diet results in elevated plasma insulin levels. These observations suggest that the activity of the pancreatic B cell in teleosts like those of mammals is modified by different nutritional states particularly in response to changes in protein metabolism.

The blood glucose of teleosts is generally very resistant to the effect of mammalian insulins whereas teleost insulins themselves bring about a marked hypoglycaemia in a few hours after injection

Table 3.2: Plasma Insulin and Glucose Levels in Cod, Rainbow Trout, Dab, European Eel, Plaice, and Pike

Species	Number	Weight (g)[a]	Plasma glucose (mg/dl)[a]	Plasma insulin (ng/ml)[a]
Cod	6	592 ± 59	63.8 ± 9.3	6.35 ± 0.81
Rainbow Trout	10	268 ± 8	61.6 ± 8.2	3.00 ± 0.47
Dab	8	140 ± 18	40.8 ± 8.9	2.75 ± 0.66
European Eel[b]	11	325 ± 12	42.2 ± 5.0	1.12 ± 0.10
Plaice	4	135 ± 17	21.0 ± 4.1	0.58 ± 0.20
Pike[c]	6	677 ± 61	81.0 ± 7.6	0.26 ± 0.15

[a] Values given as means ± SE.
[b] Two-day postoperative value on cannulated eels.
[c] Four-day postoperative value in cannulated pike.

Source: Thorpe, A. and Ince, B.W. (1976) Plasma insulin levels in teleosts determined by a charcoal-separation radioimmunoassay technique. *Gen. Comp. Endocrinol., 30*, 332-9.

of relatively low doses (Figure 3.8). These doses may still be in the pharmacological range. Insulin in teleosts may not play an important part in glucose homeostasis. For instance oral glucose tests, a diagnostic procedure used in the detection of human diabetes, indicate in teleosts a persistent hyperglycaemia over a period of several hours. The plasma glucose concentration which is about 50-60 mg/100 ml in teleosts does not return to normal for five to six hours after glucose injection. This may indicate a diabetic-like state or it is more likely that a rapid glucose metabolic response is not one that a teleost in its natural state calls upon insulin to modulate. However, glucose does stimulate insulin release in the cannulated silver eel, *Anguilla anguilla.* The release is dose dependent over a range of glucose loads from 10 to 100 mg/kg but higher doses produce no greater increments than 100 mg/kg.

As mentioned earlier although the effects of the drug alloxan has a variable effect on the B cell cytology its hyperglycaemic (and toxic) effects in teleosts are well marked. Alloxan injected intra-arterially (50-100 mg/kg) into the Northern Pike, *Esox lucius*, results in hyperglycaemia which returns to normal within 24 hours. Streptozotocin at the same dosage does not alter blood glucose concentration in this fish.

Although insulin appears to play little part in glucose homeostasis in fish there is a reasonable amount of evidence linking its action to amino acid metabolism. Some years ago it was shown in the toadfish, *Opsanus tau*, that insulin accelerated the incorporation of radioactive glycine into skeletal muscle protein. Other amino acids have been shown to be incorporated into the skeletal muscle of other teleosts. These findings suggest that one of the primary effects of insulin is on the incorporation of amino acids into skeletal muscle. Teleost insulins cause a reduction in plasma amino acid nitrogen as do mammalian insulins (Figure 3.8). Furthermore, protein turnover in the carp liver is significantly reduced by insulin; the half-life of tritiated protein in the liver is increased to twice the control value.

Amino acids also stimulate insulin release. Arginine and lysine injections of 10, 25 and 100 mg/kg cause greater significant increases in the plasma insulin levels of the eel than glucose at the same dose levels. Lysine, leucine and phenylalanine stimulate biphasic insulin secretion from the perfused eel pancreas (Figure 3.9). Arginine also elicits a biphasic pattern of insulin release in this fish but does not stimulate insulin release at all in the toad fish.

Figure 3.8: The Effect of a Single Intravascular Injection of Bovine and Cod Insulins (2 IU/kg) on Plasma (a) Glucose, (b) Cholesterol and (c) Amino Acid Nitrogen, of the Eel, *Anguilla anguilla*. Bovine insulin, open squares; codfish insulin, open triangles; controls, solid circles.

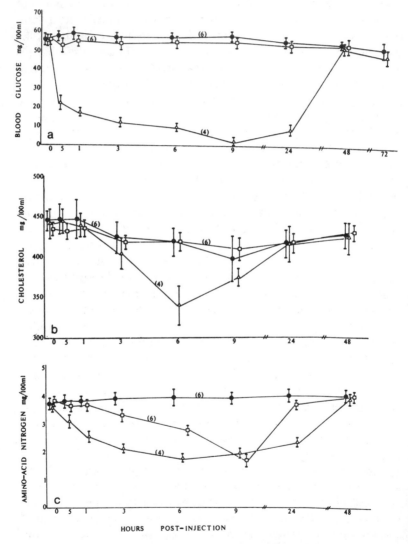

Source: Thorpe, A. (1976) Studies on the roles of insulin in teleost metabolism. In T. Grillo, L. Liebson and A. Epple (eds.), *The Evolution of Pancreatic Islets*. Pergamon, Oxford.

Figure 3.9: Effects of 10m*M* L-Lysine (●), L-Leucine (■), L-Phenylalanine (▲), and L-Histidine (○) on Insulin Secretion from the Perfused Eel Pancreas. Mean ± SE. Number of perfusions in parentheses. Temperature = 21°C. The insulin secretory response to lysine, leucine, and phenylalanine is biphasic, the peak concentrations occurring after 5 min and falling to lower, essentially stable values for the remainder of the experimental period (indicated by vertical arrows). The response to histidine however is only slightly greater than basal insulin secretion. Lysine is the most potent insulin secretagogue in this series.

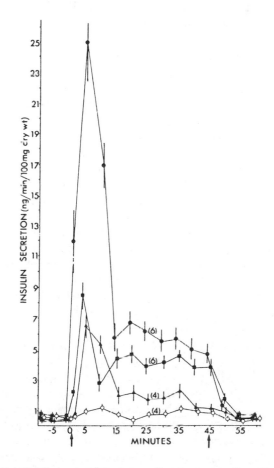

Source: Ince, B. (1980) Amino acid stimulation of insulin secretion from the *in situ* perfused eel pancreas; modification by somatostatin, adrenaline, and theophylline. *Gen. Comp. Endocrinol.*, 40, 275-82.

The natural diet of most teleost fish is a carnivorous one and it has been shown that complex carbohydrates are poorly assimilated by many fish and that glucose is comparatively slowly oxidised. Nevertheless, glucose is continually required as a primary fuel for brain, nervous tissue and erythrocyte metabolism. Therefore the synthesis of glucose from protein or lipid by gluconeogenesis may be an important biochemical pathway in fish and possibly one influenced by hormones. Gluconeogenesis from alanine occurs in trout at the same rate whether starved or given a high protein diet. There is, however, a lower rate of liver gluconeogenesis in trout when fed a high carbohydrate-low protein diet. The gluconeogenesis both in starved trout and in trout given a low protein diet is significantly decreased by insulin. The enzymes phosphoenolpyruvate carboxykinase and pyruvate kinase are reduced by insulin in trout fed a high protein diet. This inhibition of gluconeogenic and glucose utilisation enzyme activity may be the manner in which blood glucose concentration is regulated in teleosts and is possibly related to the protein conserving hypoaminoacidaemic action of insulin in this group of vertebrates.

Isletectomy, or removal of the Brockmann bodies, can be performed in teleost fish particularly in species such as *Cottus scorpius* and *Lophius piscatorius* where the bodies are concentrated into one or two discrete tissue masses. A criticism of isletectomy is always, however, the fact that residual masses of endocrine pancreas may still remain in the animal unless a complete histological scan is made of the viscera. Nevertheless this operation has been made on a number of teleosts inducing a diabetic state with hyperglycaemia and glycosuria (Figure 3.10). Isletectomy has also been reported to cause a decrease in serum cholesterol levels, a result in marked contrast to the effect of insulin injection which also results in lowered cholesterol levels in the eel.

The removal of the whole pancreas of the eel, *Anguilla rostrata*, results in little or no change in glucose concentration in the blood. However, while the pancreatectomised eel survives well in fresh water early death occurs when placed in sea water. This is accompanied initially by an inability on the part of the fish to correct the (normally transitory) serum hyperosmolarity and also by a failure of the muscles to regain their normal hydration after the initial loss of tissue water. It appears then that in the eel at least the endocrine pancreas functions as an organ essential for survival in sea water.

There have been a number of studies on the release and secretion of insulin from the bony fish pancreas using both *in vitro* incubation techniques or *in vivo* perfusion methods. Glucose can maintain insulin biosynthesis in isolated catfish islets while galactose acts as an insulin secretagogue. Perfusion of the silver eel pancreas with glucose or arginine as mentioned earlier results in a biphasic insulin release, arginine being the more potent insulin secretagogue.

In teleost fish the administration of mammalian glucagon generally elicits a hyperglycaemia often accompanied by a decrease or no change in liver glycogen concentrations. In mammals the drug 3-mercaptopicolinic acid (MPA) has been shown to inhibit specifically phosphoenolpyruvate carboxykinase (PEPCK), a key

Figure 3.10: Effect of Isletectomy on the Blood Glucose Level (mg%) of *Channa punctatus*. The upper curve denotes values of the isletectomised fish and the lower of the sham-operated control fish. Vertical bars represent two standard errors of the mean.

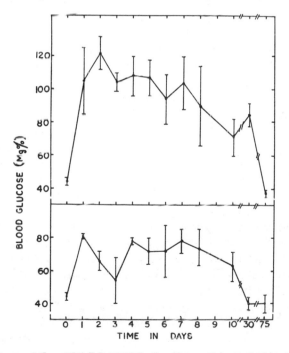

Source: Khanna, S.S. and Gill, T.S. (1972) Further observations on the blood glucose level in *Channa punctatus* (Bloch.). *Acta Zoologica*, 53, 127-33.

enzyme in regulating the synthesis of carbohydrates from the metabolic precursors of pyruvate and oxaloacetate. This drug has also been shown in the carp to inhibit the hyperglycaemic action of injected mammalian glucagon (Figure 3.11). Liver glycogen phosphorylase activity is stimulated by glucagon resulting in glycogenolysis and glucose release. However, glucagon effects in fishes appear more related to stimulation of gluconeogenesis, probably from muscle amino acids. Also glucagon depresses plasma amino nitrogen levels in the eel by stimulating hepatic amino acid incorporation from the plasma.

Figure 3.11: Effect of Glucagon (G; 0.2 mg/100 g) and/or 3-Mercaptopicolinic Acid (MPA; 10 mg/100 g) on Plasma Glucose Level in Carp. Comparison with controls (C, open circles). Each plot represents means values ± SEM (h = 4). The effect is inhibited by MPA.

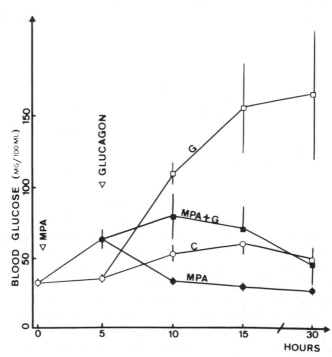

Source: Murat, J.C. *et al.* (1978) Inhibition of gluconeogenesis and glucagon-induced hyperglycemia in carp (*Cyprinus carpio* L.) *Gen. Comp. Endocrinol.*, *34*, 243-6.

Glucagon injection in mammals has been shown to be insulinotropic and a similar phenomenon has been observed in the lamprey. However, in the eel although mammalian glucagon (50 mg/kg) results in rapid hyperglycaemia no increase in insulin secretion occurs.

Somatostatin

Evidence for both the existence and the biological role of somatostatin in cyclostomes and fishes is scanty. Immunoreactive somatostatin has been identified in *Lampetra fluviatilis* islet lobules and hagfish islet organs, intestinal mucosa and brain in comparable concentrations. However, the somatostatin content of the hagfish islet organ is greater than the somatostatin content of the rat pancreas. Incubation of hagfish islet organs in synthetic cyclic somatostatin decreases insulin release. Similar experiments have yet to be made for elasmobranchs. A somatostatin-like antigen has been localised in the brain and digestive tract of the rainbow trout and somatostatin has been shown in the eel to inhibit B cell secretory activity as in hagfish.

The question is: is insulin inhibition a physiological role for somatostatin in fishes? Certainly in mammals somatostatin inhibits both insulin and glucagon secretion and mammalian physiologists have hypothesised a direct controlling relationship between the A, B and D cells of the endocrine pancreas.

Gastrointestinal Hormones

The gastrointestinal tract of vertebrate animals is the site of production and release of many hormones some of which act solely on the gastrointestinal organs themselves and some which act on all organs of the body. A number of presumptive hormones have been identified whose physiological role has yet to be determined. The regulation of gastric and pancreatic secretion and gall bladder contraction in mammals was for many years regarded as being controlled by three hormones, gastrin, secretin and cholecystokinin (CCK) and possibly a gastric inhibitory peptide (GIP). However, during the past decade over a dozen additional peptides have been identified in the endocrine cells or nerves of the gastrointestinal tract and brain and have been shown to have biological effects upon the tract. The situation in the lower vertebrates and particularly fish is far from clear. For although early studies such as those of Bayliss and Starling in 1903 were thought to indicate that the control mechanisms of gut activity were similar in all vertebrates this is now believed not to be so. For example no gastrin-like biological activity has been evidenced in the cyclostome gut.

However, it must be remembered that many fewer investigations have been made of the hormonal control of gut activity in fish than in mammals and rarely have the four classical steps required to establish the existence of a gastrointestinal hormone been carried out. These steps are first, the demonstration physiologically that a stimulus applied to one part of the digestive tract changes activity in another part, secondly, the demonstration of persistence of the effect after nervous severance, thirdly, the extraction of a substance from the gut which will, when injected into the blood, have identical effects to the stimulus and finally the substance must be identified chemically and its structure confirmed by synthesis. This is an ideal that has not been achieved for fish or cyclostome gastrointestinal hormones; however, a picture of hormonal gut control is beginning to emerge.

Gastrin

This is an established hormone of higher vertebrates and like all gastrointestinal hormones is a polypeptide. It occurs in mammals in a number of forms with differing amino acid chain lengths and arrangements but with a common carboxyl terminal pentapeptide sequence. Gastrin was the first gut peptide for which the chemical structure was determined. The hormone is produced by the G cell of the antral mucosa in the stomach of mammals and the main physiological action of gastrin is the stimulation of acid secretion by the stomach. The hormone also has a trophic action in specifically stimulating growth of the stomach and intestinal mucosa. Gastrin like so many gastrointestinal peptides has many pharmacological effects which makes the 'normal' role of the hormone difficult to assess.

Gastrin-like activity, as mentioned previously, has not been identified in cyclostomes but has in elasmobranchs and teleosts. Using guinea-pig gall bladder and antral stomach muscle strips Vigna has been able to identify gastrin-like activity from the stomach of coho salmon, *Oncorhynchus kisutch*, and dogfish. *Squalus acanthias*, but not from the intestine of the hagfish,

Eptatretus stouti (Table 3.3). Gastrin-like activity has also been reported from the stomach of the teleost, *Lepomis macrochirus*, and the elasmobranch, *Rhinobatus productus*. However, whether a physiological gastrin activity occurs in fish is problematic for neither the synthetic hormone pentagastrin nor mucosal stomach extracts stimulate gastric acid secretion in teleost fish. Histamine, however, when injected intramuscularly into cod, *Gadus morhua*, evokes a dose-dependent secretion of gastric acid as it does in other vertebrates.

Cholecystokinin (CCK)

The gastrin-like biological effects that have been observed in elasmobranchs and teleosts may be a response to a more cholecystokinin-like hormone present in these fish. For it is well known in

Table 3.3: Threshold Dose, Ratio of Antrum/Gallbladder Threshold Dose, and Type of Biological Activity Demonstrated in Extracts of Intestine and Stomach of the Rat and Several Lower Vertebrates[a]

Standard preparation or extract	Threshold Dose				Threshold ratio antrum/ gallbladder	Biological activity
	Gallbladder		Antrum			
CCK-33 (ng)	0.040	(12)	8	(12)	200	CCK
Gastrin-17-II (ng)	100	(12)	25	(12)	0.25	Gastrin
Rat						
Intestine (eq)	0.02	(6)	2.5	(6)	125	CCK-like
Stomach (eq)	5	(3)	2	(3)	0.4	Gastrin-like
Leopard frog						
Intestine (eq)	0.04	(6)	4	(6)	100	CCK-like
Stomach (eq)	11	(2)	8	(2)	0.73	Gastrin-like
Coho salmon						
Intestine (eq)	0.015	(6)	2.2	(6)	146.6	CCK-like
Stomach (eq)	3.5	(2)	2.3	(6)	0.66	Gastrin-like
Dogfish						
Intestine (eq)	0.08	(6)	1.2	(6)	15	CCK-like
Stomach (eq)	1.3	(6)	2.7	(6)	2.08	CCK-like
Hagfish						
Intestine (eq)	40	(1)	—		—	CCK-like

[a] Calibration date for porcine CCK and gastrin-17-II are also given for comparison. The numbers in parentheses are the numbers of tests made on gallbladder or antral muscle strips from guinea pigs by laminar flow superfusion *in vitro*. The doses given for the extracts are expressed as equivalents corresponding to the numbers of intestines or stomachs extracted to yield a threshold response.

Source: Vigna, S.R. (1979) Distinction between chole-cystokinin-like and gastrin-like biological activities extracted from gastrointestinal tissues of some lower vertebrates. *Gen. Comp. Endocrinol.*, 39, 512-20.

mammals that gastrin and CCK have identical carboxyl terminal pentapeptide sequences. Also the carboxyl termini are the molecular centres of biological activities for both hormones. This commonality makes functional identification difficult. Both biological assay and immunocytochemical studies indicate a CCK-like hormone present in cyclostomes, elasmobranchs and teleosts. Also analysis of the peptide from the lamprey gut and brain has confirmed its antigenic resemblance to the *C*-terminal portion of CCK.

In mammals the entire biological activity of CCK is contained in the *C*-terminal octapeptide moiety. Two forms, a 39 and a 36 amino acid residue molecule occur. The physiological role of CCK is contraction of the gall bladder and stimulation of the pancreatic secretion of enzymes. In cyclostomes and fishes although a similar hormone appears to be present in the gut its function is uncertain. For example, although a gastrin/CCK extract of the intestine of the hagfish, *Eptatretus stouti*, results in contraction of guinea-pig gall bladder muscle pure porcine CCK-33 does not cause contraction of the hagfish gall bladder. This suggests that the hagfish lacks gall bladder CCK receptors. Extracts of intestine of river lamprey, *Lampetra fluviatilis*, also cause contraction of rabbit gall bladder in a manner similar to that of mammalian CCK. Thus CCK appears to be present in cyclostomes — but probably does not physiologically evoke gall bladder contraction. It may, however, result in pancreatic enzyme release for lipase is released from the hagfish intestine (from cells homologous to the pancreatic acinar cells of higher vertebrates) after porcine CCK injections (Figure 3.12).

Although hagfish seem to lack gall bladder CCK receptors this does not seem to be the case in teleosts. Porcine CCK or the octapeptide of CCK stimulates contraction of coho salmon gall bladder whereas other studies suggest the existence and function of CCK in teleosts. Eel, *Anguilla anguilla*, intestine extracts have been shown to contain CCK-like activity when tested on rabbit gall bladder and rat pancreas. Pike, *Esox lucius*, intestine extracts also demonstrate CCK-like activity. Indirect evidence for CCK release in teleosts has been obtained from a number of fish in which meals or injection of lipid rich material elicits gall bladder emptying. An interesting feature is that porcine CCK is approximately equipotent in stimulating contraction of both guinea-pig and coho salmon gall bladder muscle. This indicates that there has been little change

Figure 3.12: Lipase Activity (Mean ⊥ SEM, $n = 6$) Secreted from the Hagfish Intestine *in vivo*. Open bars represent lipase secreted prior to the control wash of the intestine with saline. Hatched bars represent the lipase secreted in response to the peptides tested. All peptides were injected in doses of 1 μg/g body wt. The amount of lipase secreted in response of CCK (*) was significantly greater than its own control and the saline controls ($P < 0.001$).

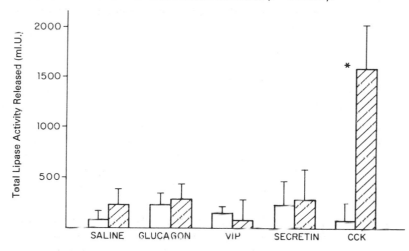

Source: Vigna, S.R. and Gorbman, A. (1979) Stimulation of intestinal lipase secretion by porcine cholecystokinin in the hagfish, *Eptatretus stouti*. Gen. Comp. Endocrinol., 38, 356-9.

in the functional CCK-gall bladder axis since the bony fish and tetrapod evolutionary lines diverged.

Mammals, birds and reptiles are known to produce gastrin and CCK as separate hormones in separate cells. From what has been previously indicated and from immunocytochemical studies in fish there would appear to be only one type of cell which secretes a gastrin/CCK-like hormone.

Secretin

While the gastrins and CCK form one family of gastrointestinal hormones there is a second large family of peptides comprising in mammals glucagon, secretin, vasoactive intestinal polypeptide (VIP) and the gastric inhibiting peptide (GIP). The molecular structure of these four peptides is closely related particularly at the *N*-terminal end of the molecule, but the relationship is not as marked as between gastrin and CCK. Secretin is a linear peptide containing 27 amino acid residues but its structure has been determined only in the pig. In mammals when acidic gastric juice is emptied into the stomach and contacts the mucosal lining of the duodenum there is a secretory response of the pancreas producing copious volumes of alkaline pancreatic digestive juice. The blood-borne mediator of this pancreatic response to acid in the intestine is the hormone secretin. This was the first hormone to be discovered by Bayliss and Starling in 1902. In fact in a publication of 1903 Bayliss and Starling prepared active extracts of 'secretin' from salmon, dogfish and skate intestine. Since this time crude extracts have been prepared from cyclostomes, holocephali, elasmobranchs and teleosts and have been shown to stimulate the flow of pancreatic juice in mammals. However, these extracts were also found to stimulate pancreatic enzyme secretion and to induce gall bladder contraction so probably they contained a cholecystokinin-like factor as well. As CCK and secretin in mammals potentiates each other's action on the pancreas precise analysis of an extract containing both hormones is difficult. Purified pike, *Esox lucius*, 'secretin' has been obtained which stimulates the rate of pancreatic juice flow but not the rate of enzyme secretion in the turkey. Whereas the response to porcine secretin is similar in this bird when assayed in rat, pike 'secretin' extract only causes a small increase in the flow of pancreatic juice compared to porcine secretin (Figure 3.13). The vasoactive intestinal polypeptide of mammals is a fairly weak stimulant of the flow of pancreatic juice in mammals themselves but a relatively strong stimulant in birds. Thus pike 'secretin' may resemble VIP more closely than porcine secretin.

Attempts to immunostain secretin cells in fish and cyclostomes have not been successful using antibodies to mammalian secretin. However, secretin-like immunostaining has been found in the cells of the stomach of a tunicate, *Styela clava*.

Figure 3.13: Dose-response Relationships for the Action of Pike Intestinal Extract and Porcine Secretin on the Rate of Flow of Juice and Rate of Protein Secretion from the Pancreas in Anaesthetised Rats. Each dose given once in random order to each of 6 animals. Responses are expressed as the peak rate of secretion which occurred in a 5-min (flow) or 10-min (protein) period after the injection.

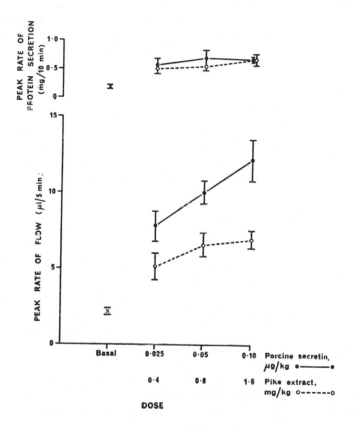

Source: Dockray, G.J. (1974) Extraction of a secretin-like factor from the intestines of pike (*Esox lucius*). *Gen. Comp. Endocrinol., 23*, 340-7.

THE 'ADRENAL' AND THE KIDNEY HORMONES

The adrenals of mammals, as the name implies, lie close to the kidneys but they are, as is well known, composed of two different tissues, the outer cortex and the inner medulla. These two tissues are in reality two distinct endocrine glands having different embryological origins and producing in amphibia, reptiles, birds and mammals different hormones. These two tissues, the chromaffin and cortical tissue, are in most vertebrates closely apposed and form a discrete organ. In fish, however, these tissues although associated with the kidney region are anatomically separated. Thus there is no 'adrenal gland' in fish but only chromaffin tissue and cortical tissue. The cortical tissue in fishes sometimes lies between the kidneys and is, therefore, often known as the 'interrenal' body or bodies or sometimes as the interrenal gland.

Chromaffin Tissue

The medullary cells of mammal adrenals stain brown with bichromate solution and green with a weak solution of ferric chloride, hence the term chromaffin tissue. These cells produce the catecholamines, adrenaline and noradrenaline and all vertebrates and many invertebrates also have other chromaffin cells scattered throughout the body which may have an endocrine function of producing the hormones adrenaline and noradrenaline. The identification of the cells which produce solely adrenaline and noradrenaline has been difficult in many vertebrates because in addition to these two hormones other tyrosine derivatives, dopamine, dopa and serotonin also form coloured precipitates after oxidation with potassium bichromate.

Cyclostomes

In the cyclostomes the chromaffin cells are dispersed in the wall of the sinus venosus along the cardinal veins and between the muscle fibres of the heart. The chromaffin cells of the lamprey heart have been studied by the Hillarp-Falck fluorescence-histochemical method for monoamines. Cells which show a green or yellow-green fluorescence after treatment with formaldehyde are numerous in the sinus venosus and atrium being localised on the surface of the muscle bundles. In the sinus venosus they form a continuous layer covering the internal surface. Electron microscope studies show the cytoplasm of these cells to contain numerous granules with a size of 1,000-3,000 Å (100-300 nm) which are surrounded by a membrane of about 50 Å (5 nm) thickness. Granules of a similar type also occur in the chromaffin cells of the hagfish heart.

The heart and surrounding vessels of cyclostomes contain relatively large amounts of adrenaline and noradrenaline. In *Myxine glutinosa* there is more adrenaline in the ventricle and more noradrenaline in the atrium while in *Lampetra fluviatilis* it is the atrium which contains nearly all adrenaline. The reason for this is unknown. The formation of adrenaline from noradrenaline with the aid of the enzyme phenylethanolamine-N-methyl transferase takes place in cyclostomes as in all other vertebrate chromaffin tissue. The catecholamines produced by the heart and heart vessels are probably continually released into the blood and may be increased during stress for it has been shown that lampreys with skin lesions have higher noradrenaline and adrenaline levels in the blood. The noradrenaline level was increased by a factor of twenty. In the higher vertebrates and also in the elasmobranchs and teleosts adrenaline and noradrenaline stimulate the heart, adrenaline particularly increasing heart rate and cardiac output. However, this effect is very weak or absent in cyclostomes. Nothing is known of the role, if any, played by adrenaline and noradrenaline in the physiological control of carbohydrate metabolism in cyclostomes. There is no hyperglycaemic response to stress in cyclostomes and that response which occurs a few hours after a stress stimulus may be due to corticosteroid intervention.

Chondrichthyes

In the elasmobranchs the chromaffin tissue occurs as small paired-segmentally arranged bodies lying along the medial borders of the kidney. The most anterior of these bodies in the region of the oesophagus tend to fuse (Figure 4.1). The tissue has profuse sympathetic nerve innervation. As in the cyclostomes the chromaffin tissue is quite separate from the interrenal bodies, therefore extracts of each component can be made without contamination of the other part. Large quantities of both adrenaline and noradrenaline have been found to be contained in the chromaffin tissue of elasmobranchs and also substantial amounts of the hormones are contained in the kidneys.

Extracts of chromaffin tissue from dogfish produce a marked increase in the amplitude of the heart beat in this animal and also a slight increase in frequency. Adrenaline has a similar effect. Whether this is a pharmacological effect or whether these hormones play an important physiological role in maintaining heart function can only at present be conjecture. However, there does seem to be good evidence that both hormones cause vasodilatation in the dogfish gill and that plasma from stressed dogfish contains sufficient catecholamine to produce a vasodilatory response. It seems, therefore, in elasmobranchs that circulating levels of catecholamines can play an important part in controlling branchial circulation and the decrease in vascular resistance that might be produced during stress could be of great physiological importance.

It does seem that catecholamine hormones also have an established part to play in carbohydrate metabolism. Prolonged hyperglycaemia occurs in elasmobranchs when relatively small doses of adrenaline are injected. There is also a decrease in both liver and muscle glycogen levels. The ray, *Raia erinacea*, becomes hyperglycaemic within two hours following the injection of 10-50 μg/kg body weight of adrenaline. This response is dose dependent in the dogfish, *Scyliorhinus stellaris*, where plasma glucose levels are elevated within fifteen minutes of intra-aortic infusion of the hormone. This increase is accompanied by other changes such as a rise in haematocrit levels, an increase in gill movement and an increase in aortic blood pressure. The physiological significance of noradrenaline in carbohydrate metabolism is not so definite for there are some reports of this hormone having no effect on blood glucose levels whereas some other reports indicate that noradrenaline does indeed elevate blood sugar but not as much as adrenaline. The responses that have been observed in elasmobranchs are much the same as those seen in higher vertebrates and indicate that in this group of animals these hormones represent a mechanism for enabling them to react rapidly to stress in their environment.

Catecholamines stimulate lipolysis in mammalian adipose tissue and this appears to occur in elasmobranchs. In the nurse shark, *Ginglymostoma cirratum*, adrenaline and noradrenaline both decrease the incorporation of [1-^{14}C]acetate into the total lipids

Figure 4.1: Elasmobranch and Teleost Adrenal. CT, chromaffin tissue; IT, interrenal tissue; K, kidney; PC, post-cardinal vein; SG, sympathetic ganglion.

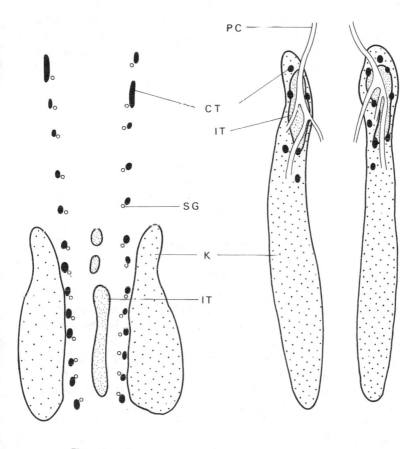

Elasmobranch   Teleost

and the various lipid fractions of the liver. The two hormones appear to be about equally effective except that noradrenaline decreases the uptake of acetate by the triglyceride fraction more than adrenaline. As elasmobranchs have high levels of plasma catecholamines, for example, estimates give *Scyliorhinus canicula* as having plasma levels of 1-8 μg/100ml adrenaline and plasma levels of 2-14 μg/100ml of noradrenaline, then it would be expected that their excretion rate would be rapid. This is indeed the case and the rate of catecholamine deactivation and excretion is comparable to that of mammals although their body temperature is much lower. The biochemical pathway for breakdown is the same as in the higher vertebrates namely by deamination and *O*-methylation. Metanephrine, normetanephrine and 3-methoxy-4-hydroxymandelic acid are the main metabolites produced. This is in contrast to teleosts where only metanephrine has been identified as a metabolite of adrenaline.

Osteichthyes

The chromaffin tissue of the lungfish, *Protopterus*, lies in the walls of the intercostal branches of the dorsal aorta. The chromaffin cell has yellowish homogeneous cytoplasm without granulation. In some cases it forms a ring around the nucleus while in other cases the main cytoplasmic mass is assymetrical to the nucleus and prolonged into strands pointing towards the lumen of the artery. These cells are innervated by sympathetic nerves in a similar manner to that of elasmobranch chromaffin tissue. The physiology of catecholamines in dipnoi is unknown.

The distribution of chromaffin tissue in teleosts varies with species as does the cytology of the tissue. However, patches of chromaffin tissue are generally found in the region of the post-cardinal venous drainage of the kidney. Sometimes the chromaffin tissue situated along the postcardinal veins is closely associated with the interrenal tissue. Nandi has classified the distribution of chromaffin tissue. In some teleosts chromaffin cells are embedded in the vein walls and may either be or not be associated with renal tissue (Nandi type 1 and 2). In other species chromaffin tissue is always and only associated with interrenal tissue (Nandi type 3) while in two other classes (Nandi type 4 and 5) chromaffin tissue can be dispersed in the interrenal tissue and sometimes also in the vein walls. The primitive location of chromaffin tissue in teleosts is probably within the wall of the postcardinal veins.

Chromaffin cells are generally more uniform and rounded in appearance than are the interrenal cells and their cytoplasm is pale and slightly basiphilic. Most of these cells give a typical chromaffin reaction but this is not invariably so. Cells which on morphological grounds may be classified as chromaffin sometimes fail to give a chromaffin reaction. *Clupea* species show no chromaffin reaction in their 'chromaffin' tissue. Some of the difficulties that have been encountered in identifying chromaffin tissue are due no doubt to the variable dispersion of the tissue in the kidney region. The presence of a pigment cell in the kidney which gives a positive chromaffin reaction also confuses knowledge of the distribution of chromaffin tissue in teleosts. The potassium iodate test which in mammals demonstrates noradrenaline but not noradrenaline histochemically gives variable reactions on the chromaffin tissue of teleosts possibly indicating that in some species little, if any, noradrenaline is produced by this tissue.

Both the anterior kidney region and the plasma of teleosts have been shown chemically to contain adrenaline and noradrenaline. There is considerable variation in the concentration of these two hormones in the plasma and also how they react to stress. The concentrations are very low compared with other vertebrates and it is difficult to give exact values for circulating levels of adrenaline and noradrenaline in teleosts as published measurements tend to change as techniques of assay become more refined. A current estimate of plasma adrenaline and noradrenaline of the eel is 1.3 and 3.4 pmol/ml respectively. Stressful conditions invariably cause an increase of these catecholamines but in some species it is adrenaline while in other species it is noradrenaline that is produced in larger amounts following a stress stimulus. The hormonal response to such disturbances is rapid as it is in the higher vertebrates. In the rainbow trout the concentration of plasma adrenaline can rise several hundredfold within a few minutes of a disturbing action, for example, handling for a short time. Elevated plasma catecholamine levels decrease relatively rapidly during the recovery of some fish but in salmon it may be several days before they reach 'normal' levels (Figure 4.2). During disturbance the anterior kidney concentrations of adrenaline and noradrenaline do not change appreciably. Heart and liver adrenaline content increases in the rainbow trout after disturbance but not muscle adrenaline or noradrenaline. The most obvious physiological change that occurs with elevated catecholamine levels in teleosts is the marked hyperglycaemia. However, changes in liver glycogen have not always been detected in response to disturbance or severe exertion, but this may be a reflection of the variability of glycogen levels encountered in teleost livers for in fish which have high initial liver glycogen values a reduction does occur. Also reduction of muscle glycogen occurs. Injections of adrenaline (Figure 4.3) and of noradrenaline also result in immediate hyperglycaemia although noradrenaline seems somewhat slower acting. The increase in plasma glucose in teleosts appears to be mediated in the liver and muscle in much the same way as in mammals, that is, as a result of activation of phosphorylase due to the formation of cyclic AMP. This is similar to that which occurs in the elasmobranchs but it must be remembered that in lampreys adrenaline appears to mobilise glycogen only in the liver and not in the muscle.

Glycogen phosphorylase has been identified in the liver of the rainbow trout. The enzyme exists in an active and inactive form and the main stimulator is glucose. The activity of the enzyme has been shown to be increased after adrenaline injection. Handling stress and injection of catecholamines provoke an increase in cyclic

Figure 4.2: Effects of Struggling out of the Water, Holding and Hauling in a Net on Plasma Catecholamine Concentrations in Several Species of Pacific Salmon.

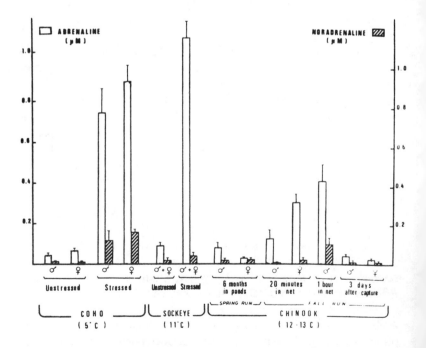

Source: Mazeaud, M.M. and Mazeaud, F. (1981) Adrenergic responses to stress in fish, in A.D. Pickering (ed.), Stress in Fish, Academic Press, London, p. 49.

Figure 4.3: Effect of a Single Injection of Adrenaline on Blood
Glucose and Free Fatty Acid (FFA) in the Teleost, *Cyprinus carpio.*
A: Pulse of blood adrenaline after injection. B: Blood glucose and
free fatty acid (FFA) levels; blood adrenaline is shown (arrowed) on
the same time scale for comparison.

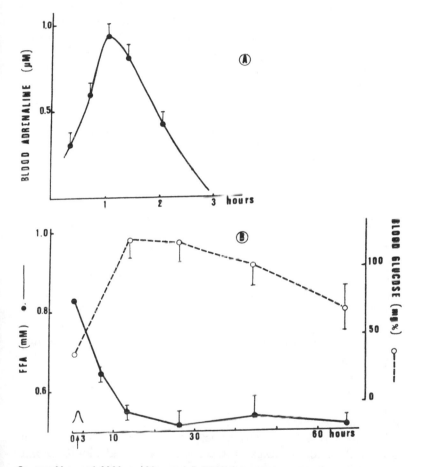

Source: Mazeaud, M.M. and Mazeaud, F. (1981) Adrenergic responses to stress in fish,
in A.D. Pickering (ed.), *Stress in Fish*, Academic Press, London, p. 49-75.

AMP concentrations in teleost muscle. Also adrenaline increases
plasma cyclic AMP levels in the trout, but the origin of this nucleo-
tide is not yet known. There is still some doubt as to whether the
plasma concentrations of catecholamines are high enough to act

physiologically on the liver to stimulate glycogenolysis. Adrenaline in mammals can also, in addition to modifying carbohydrate metabolism, cause an increase in plasma fatty acids. However, this hyperlipidaemic response is by no means general in mammals or birds. The same situation appears to be present in fish. Adrenaline increases the plasma fatty acids of the eel, scorpion fish and seabass but decreases the plasma free fatty acids of the bream, carp (Figure 4.3) and goldfish. This may indicate genuine species differences or be a reflection of the dosage of catecholamine injected. Lower doses appear to be more effective in inducing hyperlipidaemia. The lowered plasma lipids observed may also be due to an inhibited release of insulin by adrenaline. The catecholamines in addition to the contribution to metabolic homeostasis that they make in vertebrates exert characteristic effects upon the cardiovascular system. In mammals adrenaline increases the force, amplitude and frequency of the heartbeat and decreases the peripheral circulatory resistance with a dilation of skeletal blood vessels. There is a rise in blood pressure and a considerable increase in cardiac output. Noradrenaline constricts the blood vessels of the muscles, viscera and skin and increases total peripheral resistance as well as increasing blood pressure. Are these cardiovascular effects seen in teleosts?

The effects of adrenaline on cardiovascular function have been extensively studied in teleosts and it is clear that adrenaline causes a systemic vasoconstriction and a branchial vasodilatation usually after a short acting vasoconstriction. This vasoconstriction is temperature dependent. Catecholamines also have an excitatory effect on the heart increasing both the force and the rate of beat of the isolated perfused heart of the eel. However, in the intact rainbow trout and Japanese eel low doses of adrenaline have no effect on the heart rate but in Pacific salmon low concentrations of adrenaline are reported to cause brachycardia while large concentrations result in tachycardia. Thus although in general the effects of catecholamines on the teleost heart and blood pressure are similar to those in higher vertebrates there are probably a number of species differences (Figure 4.4).

Ever since Keys and Bateman in 1932 demonstrated that chloride excretion by eel gills adapted to sea water was inhibited by adrenaline there has been continued interest into the possibility that catecholamine hormones play a physiological role in the osmoregulation of teleosts. Sea water species of fish have been

Figure 4.4: *Gadus morhua.* Upper channel, heart rate: middle channel, postbranchial blood pressure: lower channel, pre-branchial blood pressure. At arrow injection of adrenaline 5µg/kg. Note the marked bradycardia in *a*. Between *a* and *b* is 30 min and hyoscine (4 mg/kg) has been injected.

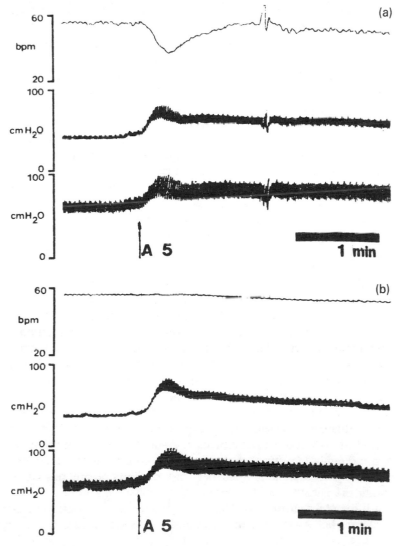

Source: Helgason, S. St. and Nilsson, S. (1973) Drug effects on pre- and post-branchial blood pressure and heart rate in a free swimming marine teleost, *Gadus morhua. Acta Physiol. Scand.*, *88*, 533.

observed to have increased plasma osmolarities after adrenaline administration. Increased plasma sodium and chloride concentrations have been reported after injection of catecholamines. All these effects might result from a direct action of the hormones on the gill epithelium either by increasing water permeability thus accelerating water loss along the osmotic gradient or by decreasing or reversing the net salt extrusion processes across the gill.

Another possibility is that these effects of catecholamines may be brought about indirectly by changes in branchial haemodynamics. For it has been shown that adrenaline increases fluid flow across the gill (Figure 4.5) while it decreases blood flow in peripheral vascular beds. The increased flow is due to vasodilation in the gill lamellar circulation taking place at the expense of filament circulation. This means that the 'chloride' cells of the gill filaments, i.e. the site of active salt extrusion in the gill, are deprived of blood supply and thus have a diminished salt excreting capacity. However, the balance of evidence favours the view that the catecholamines increase the permeability of the gill epithelium and modify the activity of the chloride secreting cells in this way rather than exerting an indirect haemodynamic effect. Various models illustrating how catecholamines (and neurohypophysial hormones) might alter the respiratory and osmoregulatory function of the gill epithelia have been proposed. It seems that a direct increase of transepithelial water exchange and an increase in permeability of both apical and basal gill epithelial membranes are the most likely manner in which catecholamines exert their gill effects. These membrane changes would serve to bring about the hypernatraemia and hyperosmolarity required of teleosts in fresh water and of the retention of water in salt water. Although stress situations disturb the fluid and ion balance of teleosts and it is highly likely that catecholamines may regulate the balance, the manner in which any released catecholamines influence osmoregulation is still far from certain. It is even less certain what role these hormones might play in osmoregulation during normal unstressed conditions. The concentration of catecholamines per unit of body weight increases during the early larval developmental stages of the rainbow trout and it may be that this increase is associated with the beginning of predatory behaviour and an active and aggressive life.

Figure 4.5: Effects of Adrenaline (10^{-7} mol/l), Phentolamine (10^{-5} mol/l) and Pronethalol, (10^{-5} mol/l) on the Rate of Flow through an Eel Gill Perfused with Filtered Ringer Solution. The relevant section of the recording was too long to photograph so the drops have been counted and plotted with rate of flow expressed in ml/h, i.e. directly proportional to rate of flow. Phentolamine when administered alone in similar experiments had no effect. Gill from 368 g seawater eel suspensed in sea-water. Horizontal arrows indicate duration of infusion of drugs.

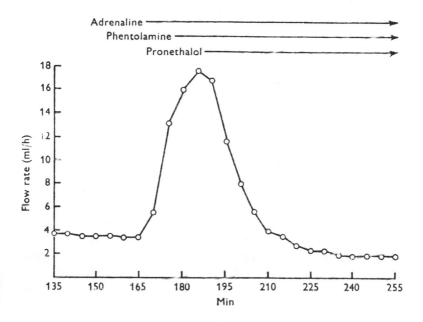

Source: Rankin, J.C. and Maetz, J. (1971) A perfused teleostean gill preparation: vascular actions of neurohypophysial hormones and catecholamines. *J. Endocrinol., 51*, 621.

Adrenal Cortex — The Interrenal Tissue

In the elasmobranchs and bony fishes cells and groups of cells are found associated with the postcardinal vessel and the kidneys. These cells which are mesonephric in origin form the suprarenal or interrenal bodies and are the sites of production of certain steroid hormones. The situation in cyclostomes is, however, confusing for although interrenal cells have been identified in the pronephric kidney and along the cardinal veins and although these cells have cytological characteristics that indicate steroid production the levels of corticosteroid hormones that have been detected in the plasma are possibly too low to be physiologically active.

Cyclostomata

In both larval and adult lampreys cells with large vacuoles and round chromatin dense nuclei are found in groups within the pronephric region on the dorsal side of the pericardium. A few of these cells also extend down to the cloaca. In the larger masses of this presumptive interrenal tissue the cells are sometimes arranged in cords as in higher vertebrates but smaller groups in the walls of the blood vessels form follicles. Little is known of any cytological changes in these cells which could indicate phases of secretion and response to experimental treatment although in *Lampetra planeri* the cell size of sexually mature animals is much larger than that of the newly metamorphosed lamprey. The presence of cholesterol, phospholipids, unsaturated lipids and acetylphosphatide has been demonstrated histochemically but attempts to localise enzymes in these cells, known in other vertebrates to be essential for corticosteroid synthesis, have not been successful. Also these cells when incubated with ^{14}C-labelled corticosteroid hormone precursors such as progesterone, cholesterol, 11-deoxycortisol and 11-deoxycorticosterone do not synthesise corticosteroids. No corticosteroid-binding protein has been found in lampreys although these proteins have been found in all other vertebrate classes. ACTH (mammalian), cortisol and aldosterone are alleged to decrease Na^+ losses in *Lampetra fluviatilis*. Recently using a sensitive double-isotope derivative assay method corticosteroids in small quantities have been identified in the blood of the Pacific hagfish *Eptatretus stouti* and in the sea lamprey *Petromyzon marinus*. Cortisol, 11-deoxycortisol, corticosterone, 11-dehydro-corticosterone were found in both animals but neither cortisone nor 11-deoxycorticosterone were found. Mammalian ACTH elevated the concentration of blood corticosterone. It must be said, however, that the functional homology between the so-called interrenal tissue of cyclostomes and the adrenal cortex of higher vertebrates is far from established.

Chondrichthyes

When one turns to the elasmobranchs the evidence for functional interrenal tissue is much more certain. The interrenal tissue in this group of fish is concentrated either into larger or smaller masses on the median surface of the kidneys or into a single well-defined organ lying between the kidneys. The shape of this organ can vary. It can be rod shaped, as in the dogfish and sharks. It can be horseshoe shaped, i.e. two elongated masses medial to each kidney connected by a band of tissue, as in the rays. It can also be 'concentrated' into a single ovoid structure as in *Torpedo* (Figure 4.1).

The histology of the interrenal in this group of fishes consists of a homogenous mass of cells grouped into cords or lobules. The cells are rounded or polygonal with a prominent nucleus and nucleolus and a cytoplasm which is much vacuolated. With lipid stains many fat and cholesterol droplets are seen in the cytoplasm. The enzyme $\Delta^5-3\beta$-hydroxysteroid dehydrogenase has been identified in the cytoplasm indicating the possibility of corticosteroidogenesis. Electron-microscope studies indicate also the possibility of more than one type of cell in the interrenal.

Although as mentioned in Chapter 1 an elasmobranch ACTH has been identified chemically its effects on interrenal histology are slight and this has given rise to the view that interrenal function in this group is somewhat independent of pituitary function.

The principal corticosteroid of the elasmobranch interrenal is 1α-hydroxycorticosterone. This steroid has not been identified in other groups of vertebrates and although this is the major steroid 11-deoxycorticosterone, 11-dehydrocorticosterone and corticosterone have all been detected in small amounts in the plasma of these fish. It has now been clearly established that cortisol and cortisone once thought to be present in elasmobranch plasma cannot be found and it must be presumed that these steroids are not secreted by the interrenals. Also the presence of aldosterone in the elasmobranch interrenal has yet to be rigorously proved.

Interrenalectomy is a difficult operation in most groups of vertebrates and elasmobranchs are no exception. The operation has been performed but with equivocal results. A slight decrease in plasma calcium has been observed but the changes in other electrolytes are often as great in sham-operated animals as in interrenalectomised. However, removal of interrenal tissue does reduce the secretory rate of fluid from the rectal gland of the skate *Raia ocellata* and injections of 1α-hydroxycorticosterone return the fluid secretion rate to normal. It is here, then, that the role of corticosteroids in elasmobranch fluid/electrolyte balance lies but the picture is far from clear. Recently though a glycoprotein which binds to 1α-hydroxycorticosterone has been isolated from skate gill cytosol and also from liver and rectal gland. The discovery of this receptor may well indicate an osmoregulatory role for elasmobranch corticosteroids.

In higher vertebrates the gluconeogenic effect of corticosteroids utilising protein or carbohydrates as substrate is well known. In elasmobranchs although interrenalectomy has no effect on liver glycogen stores corticosteroids injections do increase plasma glucose levels. Also corticosterone treatment depletes the lipid reserves of the liver in elasmobranchs and this may indicate an important gluconeogenic pathway.

The interrenals of the holocephali have not received much attention. However, in a significant experiment, Idler and his colleagues by incubating the interrenal tissue of *Hydrolagus colliei,* the ratfish, with exogenous progesterone induced production of cortisol, 11-deoxycortisol but not 1α-hydroxycorticosterone or aldosterone. Thus the pattern of steroid production of this fish appears to resemble more strongly that of the bony fish rather than the elasmobranchs.

Osteichthyes

Knowledge of the form and function of the interrenal tissue of primitive bony fish is scanty. The presumptive interrenal tissue of the coelocanth *Latimeria chalumnae* has been identified and consists of small yellow corpuscles of 0.1 to 0.2 mm in diameter lying along and in the walls of the posterior cardinal veins and its branches. The cells are vacuolated with large nucleoli and appear to contain much lipid material. Frozen tissue material of the kidney region containing these presumptive interrenal corpuscles has revealed the presence of 11-deoxycorticosterone, cortisol, corticosterone, but no cortisone or 11-deoxycortisol.

The sturgeons have interrenal tissue consisting of yellow corpuscles distributed between the kidneys close to the cardinal veins, the cells of these corpuscles are lipid containing and give the appearance of a steroid synthetic cell. However, these cells can only be regarded as forming presumptive interrenal tissue because only very slight nanogram quantities of corticosteroids have been identified in the blood of sturgeons. Similarly in the lungfish and the bowfish interrenal capsules have been identified and their cells shown to contain the enzyme Δ^5-3β-hydroxysteroid dehydrogenase indicative of corticosteroidogenesis. Plasma corticosteroids are again low making any suggestion regarding physiological function difficult. However, in the Australian lungfish *Neoceratodus*, there is an indication that the levels of aldosterone and deoxycorticosterone are much higher in females than in males.

The interrenal tissue of teleosts is embedded in the anterior ends of the kidneys and associated with the post-cardinal veins and their branches (Figure 4.1). There is great variability in the interrenal morphology among teleost groups and even variability among families. The interrenal cells are similar in appearance to the cells composing the kidney tubules but are generally more eosinophilic. The shape and size of the cells vary sometimes being polygonal, columnar, cuboidal or even sometimes spindle shaped. The cells contain lipid droplets and ascorbic acid, cholesterol, glucose-6-phosphate dehydrogenase, and Δ^5-3β-steroid dehydrogenase but in themselves none of these substances define corticosteroid production.

In order to simplify the description of the location and morphology of teleost interrenal tissue Nandi (1962) has classified the tissue as follows:

Type I: Interrenal tissue surrounding the post-cardinal veins or their largest branches.

Type II: Interrenal tissue surrounding small or medium-sized branches of the veins and, therefore, rather widely dispersed throughout the anterior parts of the kidney.

Type III: Interrenal tissue associated with venous sinuses within the anterior kidney tissue: often forming strands or cords of cells, sometimes scattered through the haemopoietic tissue which it sometimes appears to replace.

Type IV: Interrenal tissue forming a solid mass of cells in a localised area.

Often the interrenal cells are closely associated with chromaffin cells. The fine structure of the teleost interrenal cells is in general similar to that of mammalian adrenocortical cells. The central round nucleus is surrounded by a loose outer nuclear membrane, there are many mitochondria and a moderate amount of endoplasmic reticulum, many ribosomes and a large Golgi apparatus. The form of interrenal cells has been shown to change in response to hormones, drugs, stress or salinity changes and also to hypophysectomy. This latter operation has been performed on a number of teleost fish and the results of the operation on the structure of the interrenal observed. Atrophy of the tissue invariably occurs but the degree depends on species, length of time after the operation and the environment. Generally, however, three or four weeks after hypophysectomy the cells are obviously smaller, the cytoplasm contains many small vacuoles, the nuclei are smaller, the nucleoplasm is much darker with irregular chromatin bodies and the nucleoli become indistinct. The fine structure after hypophysectomy is also much changed. The tubulovesicular nature of the mitochondria diminishes and a highly electron-opaque cell type appears, the Golgi apparatus becomes indistinct and generally the cells give the appearance of being less active than normal.

The converse experiment to that above, i.e. administration of pituitary hormones rather than the removal of possible trophic hormones, has also been performed many times in teleosts. Unfortunately neither a fish adrenocorticotrophin nor releasing factors have been isolated, chemically characterised and synthesised as in the case of some mammals. Thus only extracts of fish pituitary or mammalian ACTH have been used to investigate the hypophysial control of interrenal morphology and physiology. Mammalian ACTH injections (0.4 IU/g body weight per day for seven days) result in hypertrophy and hyperplasia of the salmon, *Oncorhynchus kisutch*, interrenal. There is an increase in cell nuclear and nucleolar size and also an increase in cytoplasmic RNA. There is also an increase in vacuolisation of the haematopoietic tissue in the head kidney. These increases in cell size and number have been observed in the interrenals of a number of teleost fish after treatment with mammalian ACTH. A classic experiment using fish pituitary extracts was made by Overbeeke and Ahsan. They hypophysectomised the fresh water minnow *Couvesius plumbeaus* and examined its interrenal tissue 22, 48 and 79 days after the operation. After this time the interrenal cells were small and flat. Atrophy of the cells had commenced by 22 days and at 30 days they injected the fish with an extract made from the pituitaries of mature spawning Pacific salmon. The interrenal was restored to its normal appearance within 14 days. Ectopic pituitary transplants have also been shown to stimulate into activity the interrenals of hypophysectomised teleost fish.

The drug metopirone (metapirone, SU 4885 CIBA) which in mammals blocks 11β-hydroxylation in adrenal cortical tissue has been shown to elicit the same effect, i.e. enlargement of the inter-renal cells, in teleost fish. The interrenal cells enlarge because the drug inhibits the production of corticosteroids and with the decline of level in the blood the negative feed-back effect results in an increased ΛCTH secretion with hypertrophy of the cells in a vain response attempt to produce corticosteroids. As expected this response is not seen after hypophysectomy.

Stress, either cold, shock or the subjecting of fish to sublethal concentrations of heavy metals of detergents, results in an increase in interrenal tissue. Also during the undoubted stress of spawning in salmon, there is an increase in interrenal tissue. As the gonads of the Pacific salmon mature the interrenal tissue increases in amount and the cells take on the appearance of the cells of the fasciculata zone of the mammalian adrenal cortex. The interrenal cells radiate from the veins in great masses and displace the haematopoietic tissue of the head kidney. Not only does the stress of reproduction and sexual maturation cause histological changes (and increases in cortisol levels) in teleost interrenals but changes in environmental salinity also result in an interrenal histological response. For example, the immersion of the smolt of the Atlantic salmon into sea water provokes a rapid decrease in the vacuolisation, lipids and phospholipids of the interrenal cells along with cellular hyper-trophy.

The presence of corticosteroids in the head kidney and inter-renal tissue of teleost fish has been known for a number of years. Cortisol was first demonstrated in teleost plasma over two decades ago and appears to be the most important adrenal cortical steroid hormone secreted by bony fish. Although cortisol is quantitatively the most important steroid, cortisone and 11-deoxycortisol are also found in teleost plasma in different species. Cortisol is only identified definitely in the kidney region such as the head kidney where groups of cells having histological characteristics of inter-renal cells (eosinophilic cytoplasm and prominent nucleolus) are present.

The capacity of the head kidney to make the mineralocorticoid, aldosterone, so important for sodium retention in most mammals, was first indicated some years ago in *Fundulus*. However, its presence as an interrenal hormone in fish cannot be confirmed. It has been demonstrated in the herring and the whitefish but in a batch of 12 goldfish aldosterone was found only in the plasma of six.

It is now generally accepted in teleosts that the head kidneys produce 17α-hydroxylated corticosteroids and thus do not differ from mammalian adrenocortical tissue but there is a limited 18-oxygenation. Both the biosynthetic pathways and the metabolic breakdown of teleost corticosteroids have been investigated.

The levels of corticosteroids found in teleost interrenals and blood vary considerably both with species and with season, times of day and with the physiological state of the animal. The Atlantic halibut, *Hippoglossus hippoglossus* has 35-45 μg/100 ml plasma cortisol in June but only 5-8 μg/100 ml in August. Salmon, both the Atlantic and Pacific, have cortisol and cortisone plasma levels which vary up to tenfold depending on the stage of their up-river spawning migration. The total glucocorticosteroid levels of the channel catfish *Ictalurus punctatus* show a diurnal rhythm rising very significantly around 2.0 pm. No diurnal rhythm is seen in some species such as the eel either in its fresh water or sea water phase while in other species such as the killifish *Fundulus grandis* and the goldfish *Carassius auratus* there appears to be a bimodal rhythm in plasma cortisol with a peak occurring an hour or so after the onset of the light period as in mammals (Figure 4.6).

The basal secretion rate for cortisol has been estimated for several teleost species and as might be expected they vary. The rate for the fresh water eel varies from 0.7 to 2.6 μg/kg body weight per hour whereas that of a marine species, the sea raven, is about 9.0 μg/kg body weight per hour.

The corticosteroids of bony fish play a part in both the regulation of water and electrolyte balance and in carbohydrate and protein metabolism. The classical approach of surgical interrenalectomy is technically difficult as will be realised from the above morphological description of the tissue. Nevertheless attempts have been made. In the freshwater eel the operation results in a marked retention of water giving an increase in body weight of about 1 per cent per day. There is also haemodilution with lowered serum concentrations of sodium, magnesium and calcium. Interrenalectomised sea water eels do not survive well and are characterised by weight loss, decreased intra- and extracellular fluid volumes and by increased concentration of sodium, magnesium and calcium in the blood.

Figure 4.6: Serum Cortisol Concentrations (μg/100 ml/g body weight) in Normal Fasted Goldfish, *Carassius auratus* L. over a 24 Hour Period. Two peaks are apparent. The shaded portions at the bottom of the figure indicate hours of darkness and the open section, hours of light. Each point is mean ± SE of nine fish.

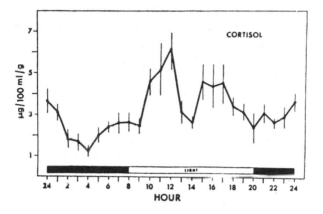

Source: Singley, J.A. and Charvin, W. (1976) Serum cortisol in normal goldfish (*Carassius auratus*). *Comp. Biochem. Physiol., 50A*, 77.

The effect of cortisol and interrenalectomy has been studied particularly closely with respect to the effect on the kidney, gill and intestine, all organs concerned with maintaining ionic and osmotic balance in fish. Quite low doses of cortisol (20 μg kg^{-1} 24 h^{-1}) increase the uptake of sodium by the gills of the fresh-water eel and the sea-water eel. The reduced sodium efflux across the gills which follows interrenalectomy can be restored to normal by small doses of cortisol. In addition to influencing sodium movement across the gill cortisol has been shown in the goldfish to accelerate branchial water influx.

The activity of the enzyme sodium and potassium activated adenosine triphosphatase (Na$^+$K$^+$-ATPase) which in many animal tissues is known to be associated with cellular sodium turnover is increased in a number of teleost gills when cortisol treated. There are some exceptions however, and the exact nature of this association is not clear.

In both the fresh-water eel and the euryhaline teleost *Sarotherodon (tilapia) mossumbicus*, when they are transferred to sea water there is a transitory rise in blood cortisol for an hour or two. This 'stress' release of cortisol into the blood is necessary for the induction of the metabolic changes necessary for bringing about ion and water regulation.

Cortisol and other corticosteroids have been shown to increase renal sodium retention and reduce glomerular filtration rate in the trout and also to increase the permeability of the urinary bladder. Interrenalectomy of fresh water-adapted eels reduces the rate of water absorption from the intestine whereas cortisol restores the water permeability.

The interrenal undoubtedly plays an important part in osmotic adjustments of teleosts and in their ability to adapt to changed salinities but they also appear to be involved in intermediary metabolism. For example, corticosteroids promote gluconeogenesis and the general pattern of their relation to protein and carbohydrate metabolism appears to be similar in most, but not all aspects, to that seen throughout the vertebrates. Interrenalectomy of eels results in hypoglycaemia and a lowering of liver glycogen as does adrenalectomy in mammals. Hypophysectomy of bony fish produces variable effects on liver and plasma carbohydrates and the very evident effects of ACTH lack seen in hypophysectomised mammals, e.g. impaired gluconeogensis, are not always observed in teleosts. Nevertheless corticosteroid injection or ACTH injections (mammalian) do in general result in hyperglycaemia and elevated liver glycogen reserves along with a depletion of non-carbohydrate reserves and a loss in body weight. The effect of corticosteroids on body protein catabolism is seen to marked effect in the Sockeye Pacific salmon when up to 60 per cent of the body protein is catabolised during the non-feeding spawning migration. At this time there is a sixfold increase in circulating corticosteroids and elevation of hepatic glycogen.

The association of 'stress' with increased plasma cortisol and glucose levels well known in mammals is also observed in bony fish. The stress may be that of handling, cold shock, anaesthetic, confinement, or scraping off of scales. All these treatments elevate cortisol levels (Figure 4.7). Thus as in the higher vertebrates corticosteroids in bony fish appear to be reinforcing the immediate catecholamine response to 'stress'. It has also been shown recently that stress exists in the social hierarchy ranking exhibited in Coho salmon. Plasma cortisol levels are lowest in dominant fish and higher in subordinate fish. Also it may be that the stress and alteration in metabolism in preparation for seaward migration causes the increase in plasma corticosteroid levels of salmon observed at this period.

Although the interrenals in teleosts are concerned with stress and spawning migration as will be discussed in Chapter 8 there does appear to be a direct relationship with gonad development and maturation. For example, gonadectomy of sexually mature Sockeye salmon results in involution of the interrenal tissue. In other fish as the ovarian weight increases so does the interrenal hypertrophy. This seasonal effect is seen in many fishes. It has been suggested that corticosteroids may mediate pituitary gonado-trophin induced maturation and ovulation of oocytes. However, here it is probably steroids synthesised in the ovary rather than the interrenals that are acting as local hormones. Nevertheless the interrenal does appear to influence oocyte maturation in teleosts and is itself influenced by the pituitary gonadotropins. Luteinising

Figure 4.7: Plasma Corticosteroid Concentrations ($\bar{x} \pm$ S.E.) in Rainbow Trout, Atlantic Salmon, and Lake Trout during the First 8 min of Confinement in a Net (R), after 6 h of Such Confinement (N) and 1, 6 and 12 h after Release from the Net (1, 6, 12). Significant ($P < 0.05$) subsets by Duncan's multiple range test are shown by bars at the top of each data set.

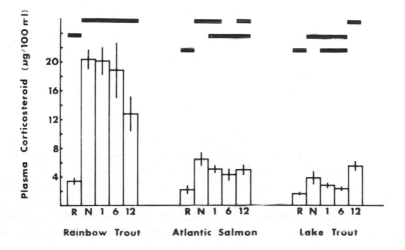

Source: Davis, K.B. and Parker, N.C. (1983) Plasma corticosteroid and chloride dynamics in rainbow trout, Atlantic salmon and lake trout during and after stress. *Aquaculture, 32*, 189-94.

hormone preparations increase the cortisol concentration of the plasma of the Indian catfish, *Heteropneustes fossilis* and cortisol induces ovulation in hypophysectomised gravid catfish but ACTH does not. Also 11-deoxycortisol induces oocyte maturation *in vitro*. As with so many hormonal interrelationships in fish this one between the interrenals and the pituitary-ovarian axis poses many interesting problems.

Renin-Angiotensin System

The enzyme renin was first demonstrated in the kidneys of rabbits in 1898. Since this time studies of the renin-angiotensin system have shown in mammals how maintenance of blood pressure and regulation of salt and water metabolism are much under the influence of this system. Renin formed in the kidneys is released into the blood stream where it acts on the plasma polypeptide angiotensinogen to form angiotensin. This octapeptide elevates blood pressure and also stimulates aldosterone secretion by the adrenals which in turn results in sodium retention by the kidneys.

Much less is known about the renin-angiotensin system in lower vertebrates but some elements of the system appear in the holocephalians and both the primitive and higher teleosts. There are also indications of a possible physiological role in teleost fish.

It is the juxtaglomerular apparatus of the kidney of mammals which is responsible for the production of renin. This apparatus consists of modified arterial cells adjacent to the glomerulus, the *juxtaglomerular cells*, a group of cells in the wall of the distal tubule attached to the vascular pole of the glomerulus known as the *macula densa* and finally a mass of cells in the mesangial region known as the *extraglomerular mesangium*, polkissen, or lacis cells.

Examination of the kidneys of cyclostomes has revealed no renal structure resembling a juxtaglomerular apparatus. Neither has renin-like activity been demonstrated in the kidney using pharmacological assay procedures. Of the cartilaginous fish the elasmobranchs also do not appear to have any morphological or pharmacological kidney features which would suggest the presence of a renin-angiotensin system. In the holocephalians, however, a renin-angiotensin system has been identified.

The ratfish, *Hydrolagus colliei* has a juxtaglomerular apparatus but no macula densa or extraglomerular mesangium have been

seen. The juxtaglomerular cells are recognised by various procedures which are regarded as indicating the presence of renin-
precursor granules (although these cells do not have the characteristic cuboidal shape of tetrapod cells). Also when ratfish kidney
extract is incubated with homologous plasma and assayed in the rat
pressor activity is observed, the activity curve of which is identical
to synthetic angiotensin II. Angiotensinogen levels are also very
low in this holocephalian. The pressor activity in the ratfish kidney
is variable and it is not yet certain if the holocephalian renin-
angiotensin system is in any way identical either chemically or
biologically to that of higher vertebrates.

Although the kidney of the coelocanth has not been examined
in detail for juxtaglomerular components granules have been
identified and kidney extracts have been shown to have renin-like
activity whose pressor curve after incubating with plasma is identical to synthetic angiotensin II. However, with the dipnoians we
begin again to get the components of the renin-angiotensin
system established. A juxtaglomerular apparatus is present in both
Protopterus and *Lepidosiren.* Granules are present but distributed
in the media of the small arteries and arterioles some distance from
a clustered group of two or three glomeruli, which are usually
supplied by a single arteriole. No extraglomerular mesangium or
macula densa has been observed. Renin pressor activity is similar
to that seen in the coelocanth.

The primitive ray-finned fish, the chondrosteans, also show
clear pressor substance formation which resembles angiotensin but
no juxtaglomerular apparatus has been observed. It may be in this
group of fishes that the source of renin is other than from the kidney.
Although extrarenal sources of renin have not been extensively
investigated in non-mammalian vertebrates it is known that the
corpuscles of Stannius of some fish produce a pressor substance
with chemical characteristics similar to those of renin.

A number of modern teleost fish have been examined for the
presence of a juxtaglomerular apparatus in the kidney. Most
teleosts have juxtaglomerular cells with granules and these granules
vary in their staining capacities from species to species. No macula
densa or extraglomerular mesangium cells are observed. Granulated cells are seen both in aglomerular and glomerular fish and in
both marine and fresh-water teleosts. In the aglomerular kidney of
the goose-fish granulated cells are seen in the walls of the arterial
branches leading to the kidney.

Renin-like pressor activity is also seen in both fresh-water and marine teleosts including those with aglomerular as well as glomerular kidneys. The renin content of fresh water teleosts kidneys is usually higher than that found in marine forms. Angiotensin in teleosts may be measured by radioimmunoassay but whereas partially purified angiotensin from the toadfish is bound by human angiotensin I antibody angiotensin from the eel is not.

The physiological role of the renin-angiotensin system in fish and the mechanism that causes renin release is unknown. However, in view of the fact that the renin content of the euryhaline teleost kidney has been shown to increase following transfer of these fish from sea water to fresh water and also that sodium regulation is modulated by the renin-angiotensin system in other vertebrates it is plausible that renin in fish may play a role in water and ion regulation (Figure 4.8). However, as previously mentioned, the corpuscles of Stannius have a renin-like activity and as homogenates of the corpuscles from a number of fish produce hypocalcaemia in *Fundulus* then possibly an angiotensin-like substance is produced which is pressor and hypocalcaemic. It is possible that calcium regulation along with blood pressure control may be the physiological role of fish angiotensins. There may exist a number of chemically different angiotensins in fish for among the angiotensin molecules of mammals amino acid substitutions are known to occur. Studies on the amino acid sequence of angiotensin I of goose fish show that it differs from mammalian angiotensin.

Figure 4.8: Changes in Plasma Renin Activity of Eels Transferred from Fresh Water to Sea Water (Upper Panel) or from Sea Water to Fresh Water (Lower Panel). Eels were transferred directly from one environment to the other and animals were killed at the times given on the abscissae. Points are means ± SEM; the number of eels is indicated in parentheses at each point. Statistical significance from grouped data analysis is given for each point. Plasma renin activity is expressed in ng equivalents angiotensin II/0.4 ml eel plasma/ 14 h incubation as bioassayed in the nephrectomised, pentobarbitone anaesthetised, pentolinium-blocked rat.

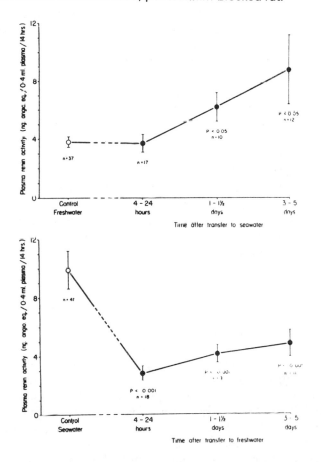

Source: Henderson, I.W. *et al.* (1976) Endocrine and environmental influences upon plasma cortisol and plasma renin activities of the eel, *Anguilla anguilla. J. Endocrinol.,* *70,* 81.

5 GONADAL HORMONES

Over a period of many years many different species of fish have been gonadectomised and the subsequent effects both on the sexual characters and the reproductive behaviour have indicated without doubt the presence of hormones produced by the gonads similar in nature to those found in all other vertebrate animals. The nature of the endocrine tissue of the gonads, the biochemistry of these androgenic and oestrogenic hormones and their biological activity will form the basis of this chapter.

Cyclostomes

The gonad of cyclostomes in both sexes is unpaired and median suspended from the dorsal wall of the body cavity by means of a mesentery of connective tissue.

The lamprey, *Lampetra fluviatilis*, ovary fills the body cavity when ripe and contains between 24,000 and 40,000 eggs. In the adult all eggs are at the same stage of development at the same time. The ovary slowly increases in weight during the winter followed by a rapid rise in spring during the period before ovulation. The female adult myxinoid, *Eptatretus stouti*, however, contains an ovary in which all stages of gametogenesis are represented. Large ovoid eggs (often over 1 cm in length), ovulated follicles, non-ovulated atretic follicles and atrophic follicles may be seen in the same ovary. The hagfish, *Myxine glutinosa*, also has no recognisable annual ovarian cycle but *Eptatretus burgeri* which lives in the coastal waters of Eastern Japan undergoes annual cyclic changes in the ovary. In lampreys each egg is surrounded by an inner granulosa (follicle cells) and an outer theca (theca folliculi interna). There are no granulosa cells around the animal pole of the egg and which of the cells surrounding the egg produce the female gonadal hormones is not clear. In the sea lamprey the theca cells often possess large lipid droplets but these cells do not demonstrate any other characteristics of steroid producing cells seen in the higher vertebrates. Also histochemical procedures have not demonstrated the presence of steroidogenic enzymes in the ovary. Thus the site of any female gonadal hormone production remains unknown.

The single testis of male cyclostomes has similar histological characteristics to those seen in other vertebrates. There are a number of lobules united by connective tissue and each of these lobules contains several ampullae. These ampullae are lined by a germinal epithelium. In lampreys this epithelium divides more or less synchronously throughout the gonad. The final stages of spermatogenesis takes place suddenly just prior to spawning. In most hagfish there is no seasonal breeding season and no regular seasonal maturation of the testis. However, as we have seen for the female *Eptatretus burgeri* living in relatively shallow water the male also shows a regular seasonal development of the gonads. Leydig or interstitial cells cannot be identified in the hagfish but are present in lampreys. Histochemical tests of lamprey interstitial tissue do reveal small amounts of the steroidogenic enzyme, 3 β hydroxysteroid dehydrogenase (3 β HSDH).

Just as it has been difficult to identify histologically and cytologically any definite steroid hormone secreting cells in cyclostomes, it has also been difficult to identify biochemically either in the gonad or the plasma androgenic or oestrogenic hormones. However, with the advent of sensitive assay techniques both testosterone and oestradiol have been identified in the plasma of cyclostomes. The amounts found though are very low. Testosterone in the plasma of hagfish ranges from non-detectable amounts to 70-80 pg/ml whereas plasma oestradiol also shows a wide range of variation with 60 per cent of the animals having levels below 10-20 pg/ml. Testosterone, dihydrotestosterone and progesterone have also been detected in small amounts in the ovary of the hagfish.

The physiological active gonadal steroids of higher vertebrates are progesterone from the corpus luteum, testosterone from the testes and oestradiol from the ovaries but although these hormones have been identified in cyclostomes their physiological role is less clear. Progesterone has been identified, as it has in other groups of fish, but there is no evidence for its action as a hormone and it is probably merely an ubiquitous link in steroid biogenesis which has attained a function only in the higher vertebrates. Testosterone and oestradiol in higher vertebrates are responsible for the development of secondary sexual characteristics and for much of the male and female mating behaviour. This is probably true also for cyclostomes.

There are no obvious sexual differences between the immature and mature hagfish nor between the male and female. In the lampreys secondary sex characters differ between species. For example, in sea lampreys the males develop a rope-like ridge along the back which in the branchial region becomes distended while the females develop a fleshy keel ventrally from the anus to the caudal fin. In the river lamprey the males increase the height of their dorsal fins and the urogenital papilla grows while in the female the second dorsal fin swells at the base and an anal fold develops. In both sexes the cloacal region swells. All these secondary sexual characteristics appear to be influenced by gonadal hormones, for substitution with testosterone or oestradiol-17β restores the development of these secondary sex characters in gonadectomised lampreys. Precocious development of these features in intact lampreys is not, however, induced by androgens or oestrogens. Immature animals do, though, show a partial response to sex steroids in that the cloacal labia of both sexes become swollen and hyperaemic but the fins remain unaffected. Also testosterone induces male secondary sex characteristics in intact females whereas oestradiol-17β induces female sex characters in intact males.

It has been observed in river lampreys that the intestine of these animals undergoes atrophy soon after they enter fresh water. Gonadectomy results in growth and redifferentiation of the intestine but interestingly this intestinal hypertrophy is not counteracted by sex hormones.

As previously mentioned in the section on gonadotropins no such hormone has been isolated from the pituitary of cyclostomes and therefore the establishment of a gonadotrophin — sex hormone axis cannot be established directly. Nevertheless in lampreys both partial and total hypophysectomy have shown a picture similar to the general vertebrate one where sexual maturation depends on the pas distalis of the pituitary. The development of secondary sex characters depends on the presence of the pituitary gland and treatment with mammalian gonadotrophin or lamprey pituitary glands restores the features of sexual maturation in hypophysectomised animals.

Although the pituitary-gonad axis is well established in the lampreys this is not so for hagfish. As long as seven months after complete hypophysectomy gametogenesis still appears to go to completion in this animal indicating independence of the hagfish gonad from hypophysial gonadotropic control. Also (unlike the lamprey) subcutaneous multiple implants of pituitary gland do not affect plasma levels of sex steroids. A third piece of negative evidence is that neither oestradiol nor testosterone provokes any change in the structure of the adenohypophysial cells. Perhaps here we have the only vertebrate where there is not ultimate control of reproduction by the pituitary.

In oviparous vertebrates the liver during the reproductive phase of the female synthesises a protein yolk precursor known as *vitellogenin*. This is taken up by the ovarian follicles to form egg yolk. The synthesis of vitellogenin in the liver (vitellogenesis) is controlled principally by the action of oestrogens. Cyclostomes appear to be no exception in their vitellogenin production and hormonal control. A specific vitellogenic female plasma protein has been identified in hagfish which as in other vertebrates is phosphorus rich and its hepatic synthesis is inducible by oestrogens and to a lesser extent by progesterone. There is also evidence for oestrogen-induced vitellogenesis in the petromyzontid cyclostome the river lamprey, *Lampetra fluviatilis*. The physiological relevance of hormonal control of vitellogenesis in cyclostomes has further been established by the detection of high-affinity, low-capacity oestrogen specific binding sites in nuclei isolated from hagfish liver. These binding sites appear to be more specific for the liver nuclei of mature females.

Elasmobranchs

The testes of elasmobranchs are paired structures suspended from the roof of the body cavity by a connective tissue mesentery while the mature ovary is a single structure of variable size and appearance.

The male sex hormones that have been identified in rays and sharks are testosterone, androst-4-ene-3,17-dione, androsterone and dehydroepiandrosterone. Whereas testosterone appears in both plasma and testes the other hormones (or metabolites) appear to be restricted to the testes and sperm. As in mammals the sperm of the elasmobranch *Squalus acanthias* contains large quantities of steroids, both C_{21} and C_{19} compounds. However, this appears to be a special case for no steroids have been found in the sperm of other species of elasmobranch, e.g. *Scyliorhinus canicula* or *Raja batis*. Testosterone has been shown to be present in the plasma both in the free and conjugated forms particularly as the glucuronide. The levels of testosterone and testosterone conjugates vary both with the reproductive state of the fish and diurnally. In the male and female shark, *Raja radiata*, plasma concentrations of testosterone are significantly lower in the evenings than in the mornings. Plasma concentrations of dehydroepiandrosterone and androsterone in *Torpedo marmorata* also vary with the reproductive cycle.

The enzymes which catalyse the transformation of pregnenolone and progesterone into testosterone have been identified in the elasmobranch, *Squalus acanthias*. However, in another species *Scyliorhinus canicula* dehydroepiandrosterone appears to be the active precursor of testosterone. It is possible that the main pathway of synthesis of testosterone, beginning with pregnenolone, passes through progesterone without, however, excluding the formation of dehyroepiandrosterone as an intermediary.

Very little is known about the rates at which androgens are secreted and removed from the plasma in fish in spite of these rates being most important as regulators of plasma hormone concentration. In mammals the metabolic clearance rate (MCR) of a steroid hormone is defined as that volume of blood completely cleared of steroid in unit time. MCR is measured by continuously infusing intravenously the labelled steroid to be investigated until its concentration reaches a constant level. When this steady state occurs it must be assumed that the rate of infusion equals the removal rate. Testosterone production and metabolic clearance rates have been measured in sexually mature male and female skates, *Raja radiata*. The rates are low compared with those measured for corticosteroids. It is this low clearance rate that is possibly the reason for the high plasma testosterone levels found in elasmobranchs. Values of 2 to 20 mg/100 ml have been identified and these levels are about ten times as high as those found in man.

The report by Woting, Boticelli, Hisaw and Ringler in 1958 indicating that oestradiol-17β can be extracted from the ovaries of the dogfish, *Squalus suckleii*, is of great interest in fish endocrinology. It was in fact, the first recorded case of the chemical identification of a sex hormone in a lower vertebrate. Shortly afterwards its presence was shown in *Torpedo marmorata* along with oestriol and progesterone. Oestrone has also been shown to be present in the ovaries of some elasmobranchs. Oestradiol-17β, oestrone and oestriol have been identified in the plasma.

As in mammals a sex hormone binding protein occurs in the plasma of fish including elasmobranchs. These protein bound steroids serve as a biologically inert storage pool. A testosterone binding protein has been isolated from the serum of the mature male thorny skate which appears to be different in its binding properties from that of the human testosterone binding β-globulin. The exact nature of the elasmobranch, and for that matter any fish, sex hormone binding protein has not been determined.

Although the hormone producing tissues of the elasmobranch gonads have not been studied as extensively as those of teleosts there is sufficient evidence to show that similar cells are concerned with gonadal endocrine functions as in the higher vertebrates. For example well-defined sustentacular cells have been reported in several elasmobranch species. These cells become densely lipoidal and cholesterol positive after the discharge of spermatozoa. Steroid dehydrogenase have also been located in these cells and their electron microscopic structure is characteristic of steroid-producing cells. Steroid dehydrogenase can also be detected in the interlobular tissue between the germinal ampullae. This inter-lobular tissue is cytologically and ultrastructurally similar to the mammalian interstitial cells.

The sexually mature female elasmobranch usually has an ovary containing ten to twenty large yolk-laden eggs and a large number of maturing follicles in different stages of vitellogenesis and primary oocytes. 'Corpora lutea' have also been described in several species. Each follicle has a two-layered theca and a distinct granulosa layer. This granulosa layer can consist of a single layer of uniform columnar cells or of layers containing two cell types, one, large yolk secreting cells, and the other smaller columnar cells. Histochemical tests have indicated the presence of 3β-HSDH activity and glucose-6-phosphate dehydrogenase. The activities of these two enzymes increase every year with follicle development strongly suggesting that this is the probable site of oestrogen bio-synthesis. The theca interna appears to be composed largely of connective tissue fibres. The corpora lutea of elasmobranchs, both 'preovulatory and postovulatory' are without a clearly defined endocrine function although in some species steroid synthesis has been demonstrated histochemically in these structures.

As J.M. Dodd has remarked, gonad removal in elasmobranchs is a severe operation because of the size of the incision required and the slow healing of surface wounds. Nevertheless, this operation has been performed but there is no good direct evidence for a relationship between gonads and secondary sexual characters such as exists in teleosts and higher vertebrates. Implantation and inspection of sex steroids, however, has resulted in growth of claspers in the male and oviducal growth in the female. The process of sex steroid biosynthesis, peripheral action and metabolism in elasmobranchs is poorly understood.

Teleosts

The gonads of teleosts are paired structures both in the male and female developing along the splanchnic coelom. Unlike the cyclostomes but in common with the elasmobranchs there are often short gonoducts which discharge the gametes to the exterior. A functional single ovary or a single bilobed testis is also often seen.

Testes

The testicular structure of most teleost fishes is a mass of elongated branching tubules with thin fibrous walls lacking any permanent lining germinal epithelium. These tubules or lobules as they are often called branch into secondary and tertiary tubules and spermatogenesis follows the normal vertebrate pattern. Although the histology and cytology of sperm production in teleosts is reasonably straightforward, the precise distribution and nature of the endocrine elements within the telost testes, as in all fish, has been a subject of doubt and speculation.

The hormones that directly influence gonad development, secondary sexual characteristics and sexual behaviour in the male vertebrate can in theory be produced by (a) cells derived from the connective tissue lying between the seminiferous tubules, (b) from modified cells of the seminiferous tubules, (c) from the spermatogenic epithelium itself and (d) by organs other than the testes. The origin of male sex hormones from (a) is well known in mammals where the modified connective tissue form the 'interstitial cells' or cells of Leydig. These cells vary in their prominence in mammals but are always present as a source of testosterone. The second source (b), from cells associated with the basement membrane of the seminiferous tubules called the Sertoli or sustentacular cells (because it has been thought that they are concerned with the nourishment of sperm) is also now known to be a site of sex hormone production and they are probably also involved in the growth and maturation of the mammal sperm.

Both interstitial cells and sustentacular cells have been identified in teleosts. However, there are two strikingly different arrangements of interstitial cells that occur in teleost fish. In one group the arrangement is of the typical vertebrate pattern with the cells grouped between the seminiferous lobules (Figure 5.1a) for example the three spined stickle-back, *Gasterosteus aculeatus*, *Tilapia* spp. and the sprat, *Clupea spruttus*. In the other group the cells occur in the walls of the seminiferous tubules and are known as the tubule-boundary cells (Figure 5.1b). Examples of this distribution of the modified fibroblasts are found in the pike, *Esox lucius*, and the char, *Salvelinus willughbii*. Both the interstitial cell and boundary cell in teleosts are markedly lipid and cholesterol positive at various times in the breeding cycle. In the pike the annual boundary cell cycle is essentially similar to that of the interstitial cycle in seasonal birds with considerable cyclic change occurring in the size and lipid content of the cells.

Sertoli or sustentacular cells have been described in a number of teleost species, for example, *Gasterosteus*, *Lebistes*, *Gobius*, *Fundulus* and *Poecilia*. They are not, however, as well developed and as easily distinguishable as in the elasmobranchs. The cells are though lipid and cholesterol positive and undergo cyclic change. In the sea perch, *Cymatogaster aggregata*, there is a seasonal transition from small Sertoli cells lying adjacent to the basement membrane in winter to a large columnar layer of lipid-containing cells surrounding the sperm mass in the sexually mature gonad in summer.

As in the elasmobranchs the enzyme 3β-HSDH has been identified in both the interstitial cells and the sustentacular cells of the teleost testes again indicating possible sites of active steroid hormone biosynthesis. In the testes of the coho and pink salmon both interstitial cells and lobule boundary cells are found. However, electron microscopy reveals that whereas the interstitial cell possesses cellular organelles (such as large mitochondria with tubulovesicular cristae and an extensive agranular endoplasmic reticulum) characteristic of steroid-producing cells, the lobule

Figure 5.1: Arrangement of Interstitial Cells of Teleost Fish.

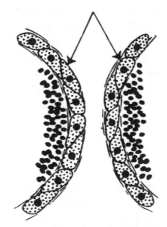

(a)

Typical vertebrate arrangement of endocrine interstitial
Leydig cells

(b)

The Leydig cell homologue in the lobule walls of certain
teleost fishes

Source: Marshall, A.J. and Lofts, B. (1956) The Leydig-cell homologue in certain teleost fishes. *Nature, 177*, 704-5.

boundary cell although having lipid droplets has an ultrastructure more characteristic of a phagocytotic function. Thus the lobule boundary cell in this case in fish is possibly homologous with the mammalian Sertoli cell.

Although the cellular identification of steroid hormone production is difficult in fish, the presence of testosterone and andro-sterone-4-ene-3,7-dione has been clearly established in the testes of the teleost, and testosterone, 11-ketotestosterone and adreno-sterone in the plasma.

Ovary

The morphological variety seen in the female reproductive tract and ovaries is immense. This is mirrored by the fact that oviparity, with eggs being shed into the water either for a brief spawning period each year or at short intervals throughout the year, ovivi-parity and also viviparity are all common phenomena in this group. The ovarian reproductive mechanisms and structures exhibited by teleost fishes can be seen in almost every vertebrate type of animal.

The teleost ovary as previously mentioned may be a hollow sac or a solid body, bilobed or single, suspended in the body cavity by a vascularised mesovarium. There may be no excurrent duct, eggs being discharged into the coelomic space and escaping by way of an abdominal pore. In the hollow sac type of ovary, however, the sac ends posteriorly in an oviduct. The majority of teleosts seem to have this latter type of ovary. The ovary like the testes in teleosts undergoes enormous change in size from a structure occupying nearly all the body cavity to a thin threadlike organ containing a few immature oocytes. The oocyte with surrounding cells form, as in all higher vertebrates, a follicle. Follicles develop from the germinal epithelium as in higher vertebrates and become sur-rounded by and embedded in connective tissue stroma. The fol-licles can develop in a number of ways (Figure 5.2) with the number of eggs produced related to the size of the egg, i.e. the amount of yolk. Surrounding the egg is an epithelial cell layer equivalent to the mammalian granulosa and surrounding the granulosa is a fibrous theca. 'Corpora lutea' can form both before and after ovulation. Atresia of a maturing follicle can occur with breakdown of the egg and a mass of cells referred to as a pre-ovulatory corpus luteum' can be formed. Or an ovulated follicle can form a luteal mass. The endocrine function of these 'corpora lutea' in fish is doubtful.

Although oestrogens are produced by the ovary the distribution of the steroidogenic endocrine tissue as in the male is uncertain. The granulosa cells, certain thecal cells, the preovulatory and postovulatory 'corpora lutea' not to mention the interstitial gland tissue have all been described as steroid producing. The enzyme

Figure 5.2: Possible Fates of the Ovarian Follicle in Different Teleost Species. cl, corpus luteum; s, scar. Ova (yolk masses) are shown in grey. Embryos develop in the ovaries of some species (for example, sea-perches), and here the ovarian epithelium and occasionally the postovulatory follicle may form a partially luteinised nutritive structure: the calyx nutricius (cn/cl).

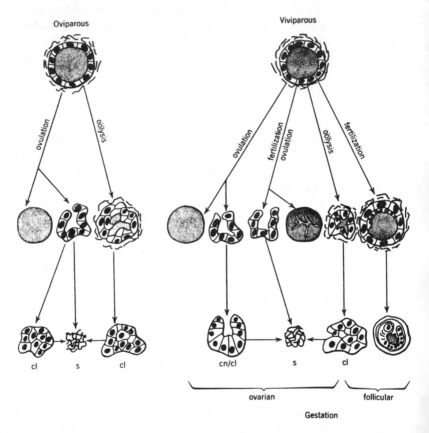

Source: Gorbman, A. and Bern, H. (1962) *Comparative Endocrinology*, John Wiley, New York, p. 260, after W.S. Hoar.

3β-HSDH has been found in abundance in the follicle granulosa cells of the viviparous guppy, *Poecilia reticulata,* but not in the corpora lutea. However, in Pacific salmon the granulosa cells do not show any convincing evidence of steroidogenesis but possess thecal cells situated near blood capillaries which have an ultrastructure characteristic of an endocrine secretory function. In a number of other species of teleosts histochemical and ultra-structural studies have implicated thecal cells as steroid producing. In some species for example, *Tilapia nilotica* and *Trachurus mediterraneus* both granulosa and thecal cells are steroidogenic.

Steroidogenesis

As previously noted a number of androgens and oestrogens have been chemically identified in the gonads and plasma of teleosts.

Testes

Over twenty years ago substances of chromatographic mobility similar to that of testosterone were extracted from the testes of *Salmo irideus* and *Cyprinus carpio* while chemical analysis of testicular tissue of the Pacific salmon, *Oncorhynchus nerka*, a few years later revealed the presence of testosterone chiefly conjugated with glucuronic acid. Following the isolation of testosterone in the testes several steroids were identified in the hermaphrodite gonad of *Seranus scriba*. Testosterone, androstenedione and androsterone were identified by thin layer and gas chromatography (Figure 5.3). Since this time these steroids together with 11-ketotestosterone have been isolated from blood and plasma of a number of fish. In both sexes testosterone occurs in the plasma both in the free form and also conjugated with glucuronic acid. 11-Ketotestosterone is not present in the plasma of all fish, e.g. in the plaice, *Pleuronectes platessa*.

Progesterone has been isolated from the gonads of teleosts but not from the plasma. Progesterone holds a key position in the metabolic pathway of steroid production in teleosts (Figure 5.4) but as it is not identified in the plasma probably has no biological role as a hormone in the male fish. Androgens are synthesised shortly after the onset of gonadal sex differentiation. For example in the rainbow trout it only becomes possible to demonstrate the enzymes necessary for hormone production at about 100 days of age. Also the steroid synthesising cytological structure cannot be demonstrated much before 100 days.

The majority of the enzymes controlling the synthesis and the transformation of steroid hormones in the fish gonad are similar to those of the mammal. However, the presence of an unusual

Figure 5.3: Structural Formulae of the Principal C_{19} Steroids Isolated from Vertebrates. I, testosterone; II, androstenedione; III, ketotestosterone; IV, dehydroepiandrosterone; V, androsterone.

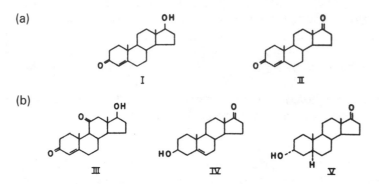

Source: Oyon, R. (1972) in D.R. Idler (ed.), *Steroids in Nonmammalian Vertebrates*, Academic Press, New York, p. 330.

Figure 5.4: Simplified Diagram of the Routes of Major Steroid Biosynthesis in the Rainbow Trout Testis. Open arrows show the putative sites of metabolic regulation.

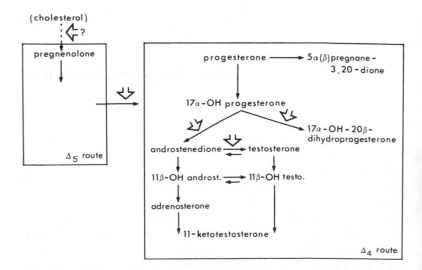

Source: Depeche, J. and Sire, O. (1982) *In vitro* metabolism of progesterone and 17α-hydroxyprogesterone in the testis of the rainbow trout, *Salmo gairdneri* Rich., at different stages of spermatogenesis. *Reprod. Nutr. Develop., 22(2)*, 427-38.

enzyme, 11-β-hydroxylase, suggests certain qualitative differences in steroid biosynthesis.

In certain fish 11-oxygenated androgens appear to be the major metabolites isolated from the testes after being incubated with suitable precursors such as radioactive labelled pregnenolone or progesterone. In other species, however, no 11-oxygenated androgens appear to be produced but this may be due to technical inadequacy and testicular 11-oxygenation may be a feature which distinguishes the teleosts testes from that of all other vertebrates.

Steroidogenesis in the rainbow trout, *Salmo gairdneri*, is both very temperature sensitive and shows different optima for the production of different metabolites. Of particular interest is the production of testosterone glucuronide (Figure 5.5). The function of this conjugate though is unknown. In mammals steroid glucuronidation is limited to the liver, and its function considered to be involved in detoxification and excretion of hormones. In teleosts as in all other groups of fish little is known about the rates at which androgens are secreted. Recently in the rainbow trout, however, it has been possible to trace the secretory response of isolated perifused ovarian fragments to maturational gonadotropin (Figure 5.6). A sex hormone binding plasma protein has been identified in the plasma of both elasmobranchs and teleosts.

Ovary

For over fifty years it has been known that extracts of fish ovaries and eggs contain substances which when bioassayed in mammals behave in a similar manner to those of oestrogenic steroids. It was in 1961 that oestradiol-17β was first identified in the ovaries of the trout, *Salmo irideus*, and the carp, *Cyprinus carpio*. Since then this hormone along with oestrone has been identified in the gonads of several species of teleosts. Recent confirmation of these hormones has been made using criteria of identity such as infra-red spectroscopy, gas-liquid chromatography, electron capture detection and double-isotope derivative assays which were not always used for earlier identification. Oestriol has also occasionally been identified. Oestradiol-17β is the major ovarian steroid of most teleosts.

Steroidogenesis in the ovaries of a number of teleost fish has been studied but a number of essential differences from mammals have been noted both in the site of hormone production, as previously mentioned, and also in biochemical pathways. In the rainbow trout steroid synthesis has been studied by incubating ovarian

Figure 5.5: Production of Testosterone Glucuronide (T-G) from Testosterone by Rainbow Trout Testes *in Vitro.*

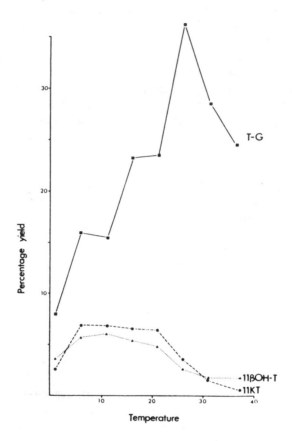

Source: Kime, D.E. (1979) The effect of temperature on the testicular steroidogenic enzymes of the rainbow trout, *Salmo gairdneri. Gen. Comp. Endocrinol., 39,* 290-6.

homogenates with tritiated pregnenolone to assess the Δ^4 and Δ^5 pathway steroids and with tritiated androstenedione to determine the oestrogen-synthesising capacity of the ovary. Pregnenolone is converted into progesterone, 17α-hydroxyprogesterone, androstenedione, testosterone, 17α-hydroxypregnenolone dehydroepiandrosterone and traces of corticosteroids. 17α-Hydroxypregnenolone increases in amount during the reproductive cycle but its role in oocyte maturation, if any, is unknown.

Figure 5.6: The Effect of GTH (50 mg/ml) Administered as a Single Pulse (a), or Continuously (b) to Isolated Ovarian Fragments of Rainbow Trout. No increase in 17α-20β-dihydroprogesterone occurs from a single pulse.

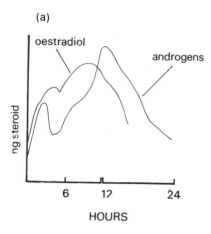

(a)

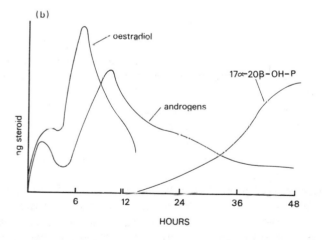

(b)

Source: Redrawn from Zohar, *et al.* (1982) in Richter, C.J. and Goos, H.J. Th. (eds.), *Proceedings of the International Symposium on 'Reproductive Physiology of Fish'*, Pudoc, Wageningen, p. 14-18.

From tritiated androstenedione, testosterone, oestrone and oestradiol-17β are produced from the incubated ovary, but the amounts of oestrone and oestradiol-17β vary in the ovary seasonally and are particularly high at the onset of vitellogenesis. This is in accord with the fact that oestrogens trigger the liver to synthesise yolk proteins.

Some of the enzymes involved in teleost ovary steroid hormone metabolism have been determined and found to have substrate velocity kinetics identical to those found in mammalian ovaries, for example, 7α-steroid reductase, and 7α-hydroxysteroid dehydrogenase.

Gonad Removal

Ablation of the gonads classically in animals helps to disclose the physiological processes and behaviour which are under the control of testicular or ovarian hormones. Teleost fish are no exception and many have been orchidectomised or ovariectomised. Castration of male fish results in loss of the special sometimes brilliant skin colour in those species with colour dimorphism. Also the nuptial coloration which appears seasonally in some male fish is affected. If castration is performed before the breeding season the nuptial colouration fails to appear and if castration is made during the breeding season the colour may rapidly fade. If only one testis is removed there is little effect on coloration, the remaining gonad producing enough hormone to maintain normal coloration. Secondary sexual characteristics such as the small dermal excrescences like white warts which appear on the anterior part of the head of the Japanese bitterling or the European minnow during the breeding season fail to appear after orchidectomy. Also the growth of the gonopodium is prevented in species showing this secondary sexual feature such as *Gambusia*.

Ovariectomy does not have the same effect on female coloration as castration does in the male teleost. Numerous experiments have been carried out injecting or implanting male or female hormones or testes and ovarian extracts into teleosts (Table 5.1). As is seen from this table the effects are similar to those seen generally in other vertebrates. However, there is inconsistency and sometimes contradiction in these effects. Much of this may be attributed to 'wrong' dosage levels of hormones injected which bear little relationship to the titres of circulating hormones. Many confusing results must be attributed also to 'wrong' hormones for often it is not known exactly what hormones are contained in the plasma and the exact chemical nature of the steroids secreted by the gonads of fish. Also workers investigating the role of gonadal hormones in fish have tended to presuppose a common pattern of action of sex hormones throughout the vertebrates and that their target organs and physiological and biological role will be similar to that seen in mammals. To a certain extent this supposition has been justified but the ovary of the oviparous or viviparous fish responds in a very different manner to oestrogens compared with the mammalian uterus response to oestrogens.

Gonadal Effects of Androgens and Oestrogens

In spite of cautions and reservation androgens clearly accelerate the rate of spermatogenesis in fish, for example in the intact carp or the hypophysectomised killifish, *Fundulus heteroclitus*, or the catfish, *Heteropneustes fossilis*. Also in *Fundulus* the weight of the testes increases after intraperitoneal injection of androgens even after hypophysectomy. The solving of the problem, however, as to whether or not the endogenous androgens in fish, as in mammals have a true physiological role in maintaining spermatogenesis is difficult to answer. However, it is probably true to say that in fish as in mammals androgens have a direct and beneficial effect on spermatogenesis.

As seen in Table 5.1 oestrogens have a variable effect on the ovary and no generalisations can be made regarding the possible sites where oestrogens might modify oogenesis or ovary structure directly.

Secondary Sexual Characters

It is well known that sex steroids have a primary role in eliciting the growth and development of secondary sexual characters in vertebrates. For as we have seen removal of gonads results in loss of these features such as nuptial coloration and gonopodium growth in fish. Secondary sexual characters are often less well developed in female teleosts but the growth of the bitterling, *Rhodeus amarus*, ovipositor is a sensitive indicator of oestrogen levels. The effect of androgen injection or implantation is also seen

Table 5.1: The Effect of Androgen and Oestrogens on the Gonads (a) and Sexual Characteristics and Reproductive Behaviour (b) of Fish.

a.i. Effects of Androgens on the Male Reproductive System of Fish

Species	Hormone	Effect
CYCLOSTOMES		
Lampetra fluviatilis	Testosterone	Slight stimulation of spermatogenesis
	Testosterone	No deleterious effects on spermatogenesis
Lampetra planeri	Testosterone propionate	No effect on testis
ELASMOBRANCHII		
Scyliorhinus caniculus	Testosterone propionate (into yolk sac)	Feminisation of testis; inhibition of gonadal medulla of genetic males
	Testosterone propionate, ethynyltestosterone (into yolk sac)	Feminisation of testis in genetic males; tendency toward intersexuality
TELEOSTEI		
Anguilla anguilla L.	Testosterone propionate	Slight regression of testis
Fundulus heteroclitus	Testosterone propionate	In hypophysectomised fish, slight testicular stimulation, little effect in intact fish
	Methyltestosterone	In hypophysectomised fish, increased spermatogenesis
Heteropneustes fossilis	Testosterone propionate	Stimulated seminal vesicle and testis, restored spermatogenesis in hypophysectomised fish
Hippocampus hippocampus	Ethynyltestosterone	Disturbed incubation of young in male fish
Lebistes reticulatus	Testosterone propionate, Ethynyltestosterone	Stimulated testis, causing eventual exhaustion and degeneration
	Ethynyltestosterone	Stimulated testis; precocious maturation
	Testosterone propionate	Stimulated testis
Oncorhynchus nerka	11-Ketotestosterone	Increased spermatogenesis
Oryzias latipes	Methyltestosterone	Sex reversal in genetic males

Species	Hormone	Effect
Phoxinus laevis	Testosterone propionate	Induction of spermatogenesis
Salmo trutta	Testosterone propionate	Inhibition of testis; accelerated development of vas deferens
Tilapia aurea	Methyltestosterone or testosterone	No effect on testis
Xiphophorus maculatus	Methyltestosterone	Stimulated testis
	Ethynyltestosterone	Stimulated testis; precocious maturation
	Ethynyltestosterone	Stimulated testis
Xiphophorus variatus	Methyltestosterone	Stimulated testis

ii. Effect of Androgens on the Female Reproductive System

Species	Hormone	Effect
CYCLOSTOMES		
Lampetra planeri	Testosterone propionate	No effect on ovary
TELEOSTEI		
Chaenogobius annularis	Testosterone	Stimulated unpaired fins in both ♂ and ♀
Gambusia affinis	Testosterone	Sex reversal
Halichoerus poecilopterus	Testosterone propionate	Sex reversal
Lebistes reticulatus	Testosterone propionate	Sex reversal
	Testosterone propionate, Ethynyltestosterone	Inhibited ovary; partial sex reversal
	Ethynyltestosterone	Partial sex reversal
Oryzias latipes	Methyltestosterone	Stimulated ♂ characters in females; inhibited by X irradiation
Phoxinus laevis	Testosterone propionate	Degeneration of ovary; thickening of oviduct
Salmo trutta	Testosterone	Inhibition of ovarian germinal epithelium; hypertrophy of oviducal epithelium
Xiphophorus helleri	Testosterone propionate	Sex reversal; spermatogenesis
	Testosterone propionate	Resorption of large eggs and abortion in pregnant female fish
	Testosterone propionate	Sex reversal; induction of spermatogenesis
	Testosterone	Induced spermatogenesis in young female; no effect on mature female

Table 5.1 continued

Xiphophorus maculatus	Ethynyltestosterone	Degeneration of ovary; inhibited yolk formation
	Ethynyltestosterone	Degeneration of ovary; ♂ gonopodia developed
Various species	Testosterone (+ PMS)	Sterile hybrids rendered fertile

iii. Effect of Oestrogenic Agents on the Male Reproductive System

Species	Hormone	Effect
ELASMOBRANCHII		
Scyliorhinus caniculus	Oestradiol	Feminisation of ♂ embryos
TELEOSTEI		
Anguilla anguilla	Oestradiol dipropionate	Partial sex reversal
Gambusia holbrooki	Oestradiol benzoate	Feminisation of males of all ages
Gambusia sp.	Oestradiol benzoate	Sex reversal
Halichoerus poecilopterus	Oestradiol benzoate	Reduction of testis
Heteropneustes fossilis	Oestradiol benzoate	No effect on spermatogenesis or seminal vesicle
Lebistes reticulatus	Oestradiol benzoate	Inhibition of spermatogenesis but no oocytes
		Incomplete sex reversal; ovotestis
Misgurnus anguillicaudatus	Ethynyloestradiol	Sex reversal
Oryzias latipes	Oestrone	Sex reversal
	Oestrone	Sex reversal
	Stilboestrol	Sex reversal
	Oestrone (into egg), Stilboestrol (into egg)	Sex reversal in genetic males
	'Estrin'	Partial sex reversal
Phoxinus laevis	Oestradiol	Degeneration of testis; on stopping injection testis recovered
Salmo trutta	Oestradiol	Inhibition of germinal tissue; accelerated vas deferens development
Tilapia aurea	Stilboestrol	Reduction of testis

Species	Hormone	Effect
Xiphophorus helleri	'Estrogen'	Decreased spermatogenesis
	Oestradiol benzoate	Partial sex reversal: ovotestis; suppression of germ cells and atrophy of testis
	Oestrogen	Inhibition of spermatogenesis, but no oocytes
	Oestradiol benzoate	Induced oogenesis in young male, no effect on testis of mature male
Xiphophorus maculatus	Oestradiol benzoate	Inhibition of spermatogenesis; ovotestis in young males
	Oestradiol benzoate	Inhibited testis
	Oestradiol	Stimulated testis in large (over 19 mm) males
Xiphophorus-Platypoecilus hybrids	Oestradiol	Inhibited testis without altering external characteristics

b. Effect of Androgens and Oestrogens on Secondary Sexual Characters and Reproductive Behaviour in Male and Female Fish

Species	Hormone	Effect
CYCLOSTOMES		
Lampetra fluviatilis	Testosterone	Cloacal swelling
ELASMOBRANCHII		
Raja radiata	Testosterone propionate	Stimulation of claspers in immature ♂; slight stimulation in body growth
Scyliorhinus caniculus	Testosterone propionate	Hyperplasia of mesonephric tubules in anterior kidney (male character) in both ♂ and ♀ embryos
TELEOSTEI		
Achailognathus intermedium	Extract of testis	Precocious nuptial coloration in ♂
Acheilognathus lanceolata	Methyltestosterone, testosterone, methylandrostenediol	Development of pearl organs(?), ovipositor (male organ) in male and female
	Oestradiol or hexestrol + HCG	Ovarian growth associated with secondary sexual changes in skin, jaws, and eyes
Anguilla anguilla	Testosterone propionate	Stimulation of seminal vesicle secretions in hypophysectomised ♂

Table 5.1 continued

Species	Hormone	Effect
Fundulus heteroclitus	Testosterone propionate	Induced nuptial colour in intact and hypophysectomised fish
	Methyltestosterone	Induced nuptial coloration in hypophysectomised fish
Gambusia affinis	Ethynyltestosterone, methyltestosterone	Induced ♂ type of gonopodium in young ♀ and in castrated young
	Methyltestosterone, ethynyltestosterone	Induced anal gonopod in female
Gambusia holbrooki	Testosterone propionate	Precocious development of secondary sexual character
Gambusia sp.	Oestrone	Stimulated and maintained gravid spot of female
Gasterosteus aculeatus	Methyltestosterone (or intraperitoneally)	In both intact and castrated males and females; full male coloration, prespawning aggressive, and territorial behaviour; in males, also nest-building behaviour
	Methyltestosterone	Induced nuptial colour in half the castrated fish; induced 'sand-digging' behaviour in castrate
Halichoerus poeciilopterus	Testosterone propionate	No change in skin colour in females despite androgen induced sex reversal (change in skin colour occurred in natural sex reversal)
Heteropneustes fossilis	Testosterone propionate	Stimulated seminal vesicle in intact and hypophysectomised male fish
	Oestradiol benzoate	No effect on seminal vesicle secretion or spermatogenesis in males
Hippocampus hippocampus	Oestradiol benzoate	Disturbed incubation of young in males
	Testosterone propionate	Disturbed incubation of young in males
Lebistes reticulatus	Testosterone propionate	Induced gonopodia in female fish
	Ethynyltestosterone	Stimulated colour and gonopod in male fish
	Testosterone propionate	
	Methyltestosterone	In female induced male secondary sexual character
	Methyltestosterone	Elongation of anal fin
	Oestradiol benzoate	Mosaic male and female secondary characters
Misgurnus anguillicaudatus	Methyltestosterone	Induced secondary sexual characters in castrates
Molliensia latipinna	Testosterone propionate	Induction of incomplete gonopod in female
Oncorhynchus nerka	11-Ketotestosterone	Increased skin thickness; decreased flesh colour (male characters) in both males and females

Species	Hormone	Effect
Oryzias latipes	Methyldihydrotestosterone, testosterone propionate	Stimulated male secondary characteristics in female fish
	Testosterone or testosterone propionate	Increase in leucophores in castrated males or intact females
	Methyltestosterone, testosterone, methylandrostenediol	Induced papillary processes in anal fin rays
	Methyltestosterone	Stimulated male nuptial colouration in castrate
	Methyltestosterone	Stimulated papillary process in anal fin rays and leucophores
	Oestradiol, methyltestosterone	Methyltestosterone induced nuptial colouration in spayed ♀; inhibited by oestradiol
	Methyltestosterone	Induction of nuptial colouration in castrated ♂, ♀, and intact ♀
	Oestradiol	Inhibited methyltestosterone-induced nuptial colouration
Phoxinus laevis	Testosterone propionate	Induction of male nuptial colouration in female
	'Estrin'	Produced female light colouration in males
Rhodeus amarus	Testosterone	Ovipositor reaction
Xiphophorus helleri	Testosterone propionate	Enhanced body colour, gonopod, and sword
	Testosterone propionate	Stimulated male colour; gonopod and sword in male and female
	Testosterone	Stimulation of ♂ colouration and tail sword
	Testosterone	Ovipositor reaction
Xiphophorus maculatus	Oestradiol benzoate	Prevented gonopod development in males; lost aggressiveness and pursued by normal males
	Oestradiol benzoate	No effect on female secondary characters
	Oestradiol	Stimulated partial to complete gonopod development in male and female
	Testosterone propionate	Development of ♂ characters in ♀
	Ethynyltestosterone	Induced gonopod in male and female, tiny sword in female, and male courtship behaviour in female
	Ethynyltestosterone	Stimulated gonopod in male and female
Xiphophorus sp.	Methyltestosterone	Induction of gonopod and tail sword

Source: Chester-Jones, I. *et al.* (1972) In D.R. Idler (ed.), *Steroids in Non-mammalian Vertebrates*. Academic Press, New York and London.

in Table 5.1; nuptial colour, gonopodium growth and fin ray growth is widely observed. A curious feature of some teleosts is that the liver during the breeding season is sexually dimorphic in structure, colour and weight. This, as will be discussed later, is probably a consequence of vitellogenin production in the liver. Administration of oestrogens to males at this time results in the transformation of their livers into the female type while administration of androgens into the female at this time results in the liver acquiring a typical male appearance.

Protein synthesis is induced by oestrogens in fish liver (see below) and muscle protein synthesis may also be induced by androgens in fish. Whether this anabolic action is physiological, as is the action of oestrogen on the liver, is unknown.

Oestrogens and Vitellogenesis

As in cyclostomes and elasmobranchs and in common with all other vertebrates teleost oestrogens are involved in specific protein synthesis in the liver, i.e. the production of vitellogenin. This protein synthesised in the liver is transported in the blood to the oocyte where it is absorbed and deposited as yolk. However, this does not exclude the oocyte itself as a site for protein synthesis and the conversion of plasma proteins into yolk protein may also require the aid of specific oocyte enzymes.

The first experiments carried out on teleost fish consisted of injecting male bass, *Paralabrax clathratus*, with very large doses (10 mg) of oestrone and observing hypertrophy of liver with much increased plasma levels of calcium, protein, phosphorus, phospholipid and lipids. Similar experiments were subsequently carried out with much smaller doses of oestrogens, a similar result being obtained both in male and female fish (Figure 5.7). This female specific protein, vitellogenin, has proved difficult to obtain in a pure and unaltered form in many teleosts. Vitellogenin of teleosts is less phosphorylated than in other vertebrates and is also highly susceptible to proteolysis. Nevertheless, a vitellogenin has now been isolated from the plasma of *Fundulus heteroclitus* in pure form. It is highly probable that a number of these female specific proteins exist. These vitellogenins are complex molecules consisting of phosphorus-containing peptides (phosvitims) and lipoproteins.

Plasma vitellogenin has been assayed by radioimmunoassay in the plasma of the Atlantic salmon, *Salmo salar*, and its presence

Figure 5.7: Production of Oestradiol Specifically Induced Protein in *Tilapia aurea*. All fish were ovariectomised after blood sampling on day 0. Oestradiol (0.5 mg in sesame oil) or the vehicle was injected on the days marked with arrows. $N =$ numbers in parentheses. (a) Plasma oestradiol levels (mean $\pm$ SEM) before ovariectomy, after ovariectomy, and in the oil-injected ovariectomised controls. (b) Plasma concentrations of calcium and total protein in intact, ovariectomised, oestradiol-injected, and oil-injected ovariectomised fish (mean $\pm$ SEM). □----□, Ca; and △----△, protein in E_2-injected fish; ■___■, Ca; and △___△; protein in oil-injected controls.

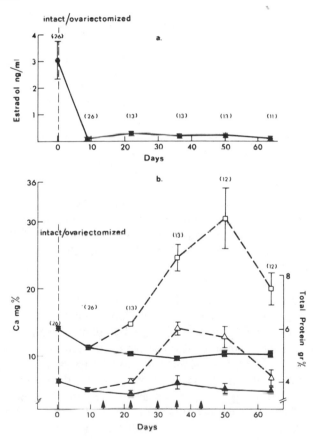

Source: Yaron, Z. *et. al.* (1977) Occurrence and biological activity of estradiol-17β in the intact and ovariectomized *Tilapia aurea* (Cichlidae, Teleostei). *Gen. Comp. Endocrinol.*, *33*, 45-52

has been used to determine the stages in maturity of migrating females. Plasma vitellogenin as would be expected varied in levels during the seasonal reproductive changes. The relationship of plasma vitellogenins to other parameters in the rainbow trout is seen in Figure 5.8. The vitellogenins peak just before spawning with barely detectable levels being present from April to September.

The deposition of yolk in the eggs is called vitellogenesis. However, it has become convenient to divide the accumulation of yolk material by fish oocytes into two phases, namely, yolk synthesis within the oocyte or 'endogenous vitellogenesis' and accumulation of yolk precursors synthesised externally to the oocyte or 'exogenous vitellogenesis'. The hormonal control of 'endogenous vitellogenesis' has not been explored in fish or for that matter other vertebrates. However, 'exogenous vitellogenesis' appears to be responsive to carbohydrate-rich gonadotrophin in teleosts which stimulate the vitellogenin incorporation into the oocyte. However, in several teleosts carbohydrate-poor gonadotrophin can also stimulate vitellogenin incorporation into oocytes as may other hormones such as corticosteroids or thyroid hormones. Oestrogens do not seem to stimulate the incorporation of yolk into the gonads of teleosts.

Calcium Changes

In addition to the changes of phosphorus in the plasma related to vitellogenin synthesis induced by oestrogens the gonadal hormones influence the movement and utilisation of other ions in fish particularly calcium. The total plasma calcium of teleost fish is about 10 mg per 100 ml. Oestradiol-17β has been shown in a number of species to cause hypercalcaemia both in males and females whereas testosterone is without effect. The calcium appearing in the plasma is either in the form of colloidal calcium phosphate or is bound to the serum phosphoprotein vitellogenin. The plasma calcium phosphate is probably derived from the scales for in both the goldfish and the killifish a single injection of oestradiol causes calcium resorption from the scales. Bone calcium deposition is also inhibited by oestrogen treatment as is the branchial uptake of calcium. The vitellogenin-bound calcium is also derived from the scales having been temporarily accumulated in the liver.

Figure 5.8: Seasonal Changes of Some Biochemical Parameters in *Salmo gairdneri.*

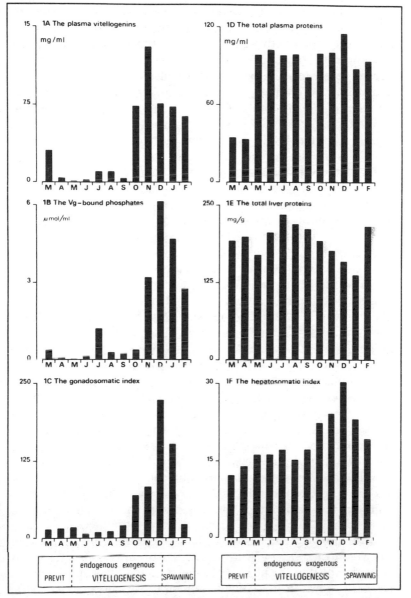

Source: van Bohemen, Ch.G., Lambert, J.G.D. and Peute, J. (1981) Annual changes in plasma and liver in relation to vitellogenesis in the female rainbow trout, *Salmo gairdneri. Gen. Comp. Endocrinol., 44*, 94-107.

Seasonal Changes of Gonadal Hormones

With the advent of radioimmunoassays it has been possible to follow the course of plasma androgen and oestrogen changes during the reproductive cycle. This is well documented for the rainbow trout (Figure 5.9). It is seen in this teleost that the testosterone levels reach a peak in November whereas the 11-keto-testosterone levels peak in February. Also in the brook trout *Salvelinus fontinalis* levels of testosterone reach a peak one month before those of 11-ketotestosterone. Again in the Atlantic salmon *Salmo salar* the levels of plasma 11-ketotestosterone increase rapidly as the fish reaches the mature stage of testes growth but levels of testosterone rise only slightly and remain at a constant level throughout the spawning and post-spawning period. All these observations suggest separate roles for these two male sex hormones. It does seem significant that the peak of 11-keto-testosterone levels coincides with spermination while the peak plasma levels of testosterone coincide with spermiogenesis. It has been pointed out, however, that testosterone is one of the intermediate products in the synthesis of 11-ketotestosterone and it is possible that the presence of this steroid in the plasma is incidental. The decrease in level of testosterone after November in the rainbow trout could possibly relate to an increase in ability of the fish to transform testosterone into 11-ketotestosterone.

The highest levels of 17β-oestradiol are seen in November just prior to ovulation which commences in December in the rainbow trout. After ovulation the hormone level falls rapidly to a basal level. Also it is seen that the female plasma contains high levels of testosterone. The female teleost ovary synthesises testosterone and converts it into 17β-oestradiol. It has been suggested that in female teleost fish testosterone may have a hormonal function rather than be solely an intermediate in the synthesis of oestrogens. Again it has been suggested that this is the way in which the sex steroids are transferred to tissue sites, the testosterone being converted into 17β-oestradiol at the tissue sites.

In addition to testosterone and 11-ketotestosterone, the steroid 11-oxotestosterone (17β-hydroxyandrost-4-en-3, 11-dione) has been identified in the plasma of salmonids and other species and it has been shown in the Atlantic salmon to vary in seasonal levels. There is a peak at the time of full maturation during October and November and again this might mean a specific concern with a

Figure 5.9: Changes in Androgens and Oestrogen of Plasma of Rainbow Trout. (a) Female fish over period of first spawning season. Mean levels of testosterone (•), 17β-oestradiol (○), and total calcium (x). (b) Male fish. Mean levels of 11-ketotestosterone and testosterone. _____, 11-ketotestosterone; ----, testosterone).

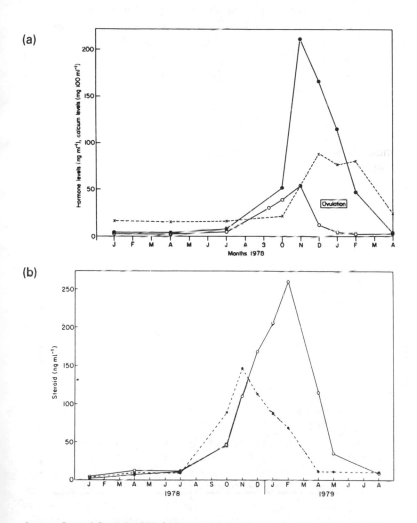

Source: Scott, A.P. *et al.* (1980) Seasonal variations in sex steroids of female rainbow trout (*Salmo gairdneri* Richardson). *J. Fish Biol., 17*, 587-92, and Seasonal variations in plasma concentrations of 11-ketotestosterone and testosterone in male rainbow trout, *Salmo gairdneri* Richardson. *J. Fish Biol., 17*, 495-505.

stage of spermatogenesis. This also seems to be the case in the rainbow trout where 11-oxotestosterone concentrations are higher in the plasma of males giving a measurable volume of sperm, the quantities of collected sperm being positively correlated with the 11-oxotestosterone levels. The biosynthesis of this steroid, apparently unique to teleosts, is illustrated in Figure 5.10.

Seasonal changes in plasma hormones have been correlated with seasonal gonadal changes in the sites of steroidogenesis. For example, again in the rainbow trout, although steroidogenesis occurs throughout the year in the stromal cells (interstitial cells and thecal cells) there is peak activity in January and February. As has been mentioned previously both Leydig cells and sustentacular cells have been identified as steroidogenic sites. The male rainbow trout have peak activity of Leydig cells from January to June, i.e. at the period when the testes are mature and new primary spermatogonia are being formed. Enzymes involved in steroidogenesis are

Figure 5.10: Biosynthesis of 11-Oxotestosterone in Fish Testes.

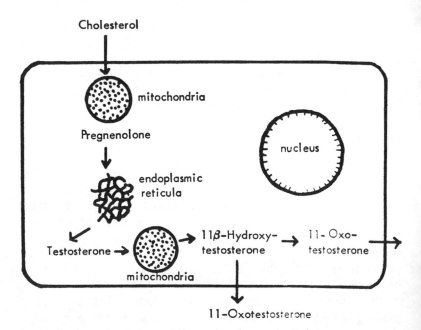

Source: Tamaoki, B-i. (1980) in G. Delrio and J. Brachet (eds.) *Steroids and Their Mechanism of Action in Nonmammalian Vertebrates*, Raven Press, New York.

present in sustentacular cells in November during spermiation.

As might be expected seasonal variation in gonadal hormones occurs only in mature fish. In the marine teleost, the plaice, *Pleuronectes platessa,* both testosterone and oestradiol-17β show seasonal variation in mature fish but not in immature fish but there is also both in mature and immature fish a seasonal elevation in cortisol (Figure 5.11). This seasonal elevation in plasma corticosteroids occurs in both migrating and non-migrating teleosts and also as is seen here the seasonal change occurs both in mature and immature fish. While it is reasonable to suppose that an increase in corticosteroids might be related to the mobilisation of metabolic energy required for gonad maturation it is more difficult to suppose that in immature fish the seasonal cortisol change is a consequence of mobilisation of stored energy to meet the changed needs of basic metabolic maintenance brought about by, for example, temperature variation. More investigation is required.

Behaviour

The reproductive behavioural and parental habits of fish are many and various and much of this behaviour is associated with an hormonal control and regulation. Although the gonads themselves appear to be involved in the regulation of sexual behaviour this regulation is integrated and directed by more direct control mechanisms, i.e. by the brain and pituitary. Also integrated into, and in part controlling, the reproductive behaviour pattern are the pheromones as will be mentioned in Chapter 7. There is also the danger, as N.R. Liley has remarked, of assuming that all reproductive behaviour must be regulated by hormones. 'It is possible that only certain components of the behaviour repertoire are under hormonal control, while other activities which are usually associated with reproduction may be causally linked to hormone-regulated activities without being themselves under the influence of the hormonal state.' Thus in trying to isolate the direct role played by gonadal hormones on reproductive behaviour one must be aware of many pitfalls.

Nevertheless, there is good evidence to show that gonads, if not gonadal hormones are important. For fifty years ago it was shown that when castrated males of the three-spined stickleback, *Gasterosteus aculeatus,* are paired with ripe females there is nearly a

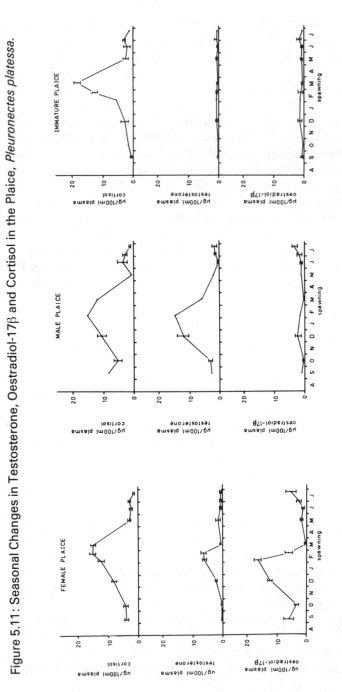

Figure 5.11: Seasonal Changes in Testosterone, Oestradiol-17β and Cortisol in the Plaice, *Pleuronectes platessa.*

Source: Wingfield, J.C. and Grimm, A.S. (1977) Seasonal changes in plasma cortisol, testosterone and oestradiol-17β in the plaice, *Pleuronectes platessa* L. Gen. Comp. Endocrinol., *31*, 1-11.

complete loss of nest-building behaviour. Also many years ago it was shown that adult castrated male salmon, *Salmo salar*, showed 'no interest' in females. However, castration does not always inhibit sexual behaviour. The castrated male jewel fish shows typical courtship and brooding behaviour for nearly a year with over a dozen normal spawnings taking place after the operation. Comparable results are obtained with male Siamese fighting fish. Similarly other female tropical aquarium fish can sometimes, when ovariectomised either retain for a long period or lose quickly their normal sexual behaviour patterns. Also *Tilapia macrocephala* continues to build nests after gonadectomy even though they have lost their sexual coloration.

Other variants are seen after gonadectomy. For example castrated male *Bathygobius soporator* do not exhibit aggressive behaviour to strange males but show normal courtship behaviour with females (they also court males and non-gravid females!). But in male *Gasterosteus aculeatus* as mentioned above although nest building is lost they continue to show a high level of prespawning aggressive behaviour, providing they are maintained under long photoperiods (direct gonadotrophin stimulation of the brain?).

A number of investigators have induced sexual behaviour in fishes by treating them with androgens and oestrogens. The method of presentation has varied and sometimes the hormones have been given to intact (at differing stages of the reproductive cycle) or gonadectomised fish. It is not surprising then that results have been variable. Generally speaking, though, sex steroids induce sexual behaviour patterns. The first experiments were made in the 1940s when testosterone was implanted into spayed and intact female swordtails. Male sexual behaviour was observed with attempts at copulation. However, when testosterone was injected into castrated male adult salmon only the 'following of the female' behaviour was observed in these males. Androgens have been used to induce male behaviour in immature female and immature male fish, but again not in all species of fish, for example juvenile sticklebacks fail to perform any nest building after androgen treatment. Also in the castrated stickleback the dosage of androgen administered in order to induce behavioural patterns is important. Low doses of methyltestosterone restore only the early stages of reproductive behaviour, i.e. digging and collecting while displacement fanning is only induced if higher doses are injected.

Less attention has been given to hormonal regulation of female behaviour probably because females are generally more passive and do not show the elaborate nest building and parental behaviour seen in a number of male teleost fish. Ovariectomy does not always result in females becoming non-receptive to males. The three-spined stickleback becomes more aggressive when ovariectomised and it may be that ovarian secretions normally suppress aggressive behaviour. Also it has been noted in these fish that the immature females are more aggressive, i.e. presumably when the oestrogen levels are low. Also oestrone injection results in a marked reduction in aggressive behaviour in the male of *Colisa latia.*

Fundamentally different mechanisms appear to regulate female sexual behaviour in different fish. It has been established by N.E. Stacey in the guppy, *Poecilia reticulata*, that ovarian oestrogen synchronises the cycle of sexual receptivity with the endogenous cycles of ovarian maturation and also increases female attractivity at the time of maximum receptivity by stimulating the release of a sexual pheromone. In the goldfish, however, it appears that prostaglandin released from the ovary or oviduct in conjunction with ovulation and the presence of ovulated eggs acts on the brain to stimulate spawning behaviour. Stacey has proposed that these two differing mechanisms are related to ovoviviparity and oviparity. In the goldfish and several other externally fertilising teleosts where sexual behaviour involves oviposition, female sexual behaviour is apparently synchronised with ovulation by mechanisms which respond to elevated plasma prostaglandins as an indicator of the presence of ovulated eggs. However, in internally fertilising species, and this applies to higher vertebrates as well, where sexual behaviour and fertilisation are dissociated in time then female behaviour is synchronised with ovulation by mechanisms which anticipate an imminent ovulation by responding to increases in plasma oestrogen associated with the development of the ovarian follicles.

Gonadal hormones in fish also affect non-reproductive behaviour. They appear to cause in several species a general increase in body activity; testosterone increases the locomotory activity of goldfish and trout. Testosterone treatment also results in an increase of appetitive behaviour. Whether these general behavioural responses are brought about by an effect on metabolism or whether the effect is a direct one on neural mechanisms is difficult to establish. Male sex hormones increase the ribonucleic acid

and protein content of carp muscle while tritium-labelled oestradiol injected into goldfish becomes rapidly incorporated into the
cells of the forebrain.

The oestrogen target cells in both the goldfish and the platyfish,
Xiphophorus maculatus are found in the vicinity of the forebrain
ventricles. This hypothalamic location of oestrogen receptors
correlates with the results of electrolytic lesion studies in fish which
have suggested preoptic and hypothalamic involvement in sexual
behaviour and reproductive activity. Forebrain ablation studies
also link this part of the brain with reproductive aggressive and
parental behaviour.

6 THE CORPUSCLES OF STANNIUS, UROPHYSIS AND PINEAL

(a) Corpuscles of Stannius

Morphology

In 1839 there was described in bony fish the occurrence of small spherical gland-like bodies lying on or embedded in the kidney. In some fish they occur attached to the mesonephric duct posterior to the kidney. They arise embryologically as evaginations of the wall of the pronephric duct. They are not homologous with adrenocortical tissue which is formed from the coelomic mesoderm. In teleosts corpuscles of Stannius can be found either as a single pair of symmetrical structures at the dorsoposterior end of the kidney as in the goldfish or stickleback, *Gasterosteus aculeatus* (Figure 6.1) or can be found scattered irregularly over the dorsal surface of the central mesonephros as in salmonids. In the Atlantic salmon, *Salmo salar*, there are about four to ten of these corpuscles of varying sizes. In a large salmon their diameter can range from about two to five millimetres. Although the largest corpuscles are seen in the largest fish corpuscle size seems unrelated to sex or gonadal development. Generally in teleosts the colour of the corpuscles is white or yellowish-pink and they have a fibrous capsule and are composed of short columnar cells closely packed in ovoid or columnar groups which may form arcs.

In the Holostei the corpuscles are generally quite numerous although in the garpike, *Lepisosteus platyrhynchus*, there are fewer. In this species there are five to seven white corpuscles occurring as round to oval structures in the mid-portion of each kidney. They are recognised as well-vascularised whitish masses projecting slightly from the surface of the kidney and are about 0.5 to 2.0 mm in size. In the bowfin, *Amia clava*, there are very many corpuscles, numbering fifty or more. It is thought that in the evolution of bony fish there has been a general contraction in numbers and an increase in relative size of the corpuscles of Stannius.

Although as will be indicated the chemical nature of any corpuscle of Stannius secretion has not been ascertained with

Figure 6.1: Topography of Corpuscles of Stannius in the Three-spined Stickleback, *Gasterosteus aculeatus*. SC, Stannius corpuscle; TK, trunk kidneys; SN, sympathetic nerve; SG, sympathetic ganglion sending branches to Stannius corpuscles and to kidneys; U, ureter; DCV, dorso-caudal vein; VCV, ventro-caudal vein; HV, vein from hypaxial musculature.

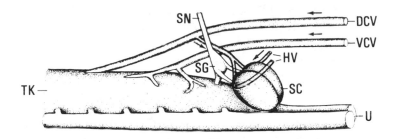

Source: Wendelaar Bonga, S.E., Greven, J.A and Veenhuls, M. (1977) Vascularization, innervation, and ultrastructure of the endocrine cell types of Stannius corpuscles in the teleost *Gasterosteus aculeatus. J. Morph., 153,* 225-44.

certainty, histochemical and ultrastructural studies have shown that the cells comprising the corpuscles are well equipped for protein synthesis and secretion. In the rainbow trout for instance the cells generally contain PAS-positive granules concentrated at the distal pole away from the lumen of the follicles which they form. The fine structure is typical of a peptide secreting gland with rough endoplasmic reticulum, Golgi apparatus and secretory granules. In addition to a few chromophobic cells the corpuscles of Stannius in the trout appear to contain two cell types, one type containing large spherical secretory granules and the other small secretory granules. The cells with large granules do not appear as active as those with small but are much more abundant in the corpuscles. In the Atlantic salmon, *Salmo salar,* and the goldfish there is said to be only one cell type in the corpuscle. However, two cell types have been clearly differentiated in the eel, *Anguilla anguilla,* and in the three-spined stickleback, *Gasterosteus aculeatus,* and other teleost species.

The corpuscles of Stannius possess intimate vascularisation and innervation (Figure 6.1) and in the Atlantic salmon, for example, a distinctive vasculo-ganglionic unit is formed in close proximity to each corpuscle. These units include one or more vessels with greatly thickened walls, tangential and cross sections of nerve fibres and two or three clusters of ganglionic cells. In the three-spined stickleback, the corpuscles are supplied with blood by the caudal veins and by small segmental vessels coming from the hypaxial musculature. A portal system is formed and the direction of blood flow ensures that the blood coming from the corpuscles passes through the kidney. In the stickleback also the corpuscle of Stannius is innervated by a sympathetic nerve (Figure 6.1), which in the area of the corpuscle shows a ganglionic swelling made up of several groups of cell bodies as in the Atlantic salmon. From this ganglion two small nerves penetrate and ramify into the corpuscle.

Removal of the Corpuscles of Stannius

With the structure of the corpuscles being decidedly glandular it was surprising that it was not until 1964 that attempts were made to extirpate these structures. In certain species such as the eel *Anguilla anguilla* where there are just two corpuscles it is relatively easy to remove this tissue from the living animal. According to I. Chester-Jones the operation of removal of corpuscles of Stannius should be called 'stanniosomatiectomy' because the frequently used term 'stanniectomy' has the unfortunate meaning of cutting out Stannius! Perhaps the phrase Stannius corpuscle removal may contain a few more letters but it is easier to pronounce.

The removal of corpuscles of Stannius in the eel results in a lowering of plasma sodium and an increase of plasma potassium and calcium. Corpuscle removal in the goldfish confirms this effect on plasma ion composition. However, in other species removal of the corpuscles has only consistently resulted in an increase of plasma calcium. It is now well established that the corpuscles of Stannius are a primary force in calcium regulation in teleosts with removal of the corpuscles of Stannius causing a prompt rise in plasma calcium levels. Treatment of intact teleosts, such as eels, with extracts of corpuscles of Stannius causes a marked fall in calcium levels (Figure 6.2). However, although in the eel the plasma calcium levels rise after corpuscle of Stannius removal reaching a high point some eight or nine days after the operation the levels then remain steady and may gradually decline to normal. This suggests that possibly another hormone takes over the homeostatic role.

Sea water is high in calcium compared to fresh water and histo-logical observations on the corpuscles of Stannius indicate that the

Figure 6.2: The Effects of Removal of Stannius Corpuscles (a) and Injection of Stannius Corpuscle Extracts (b) on the Electrolyte Content of Eel Plasma.

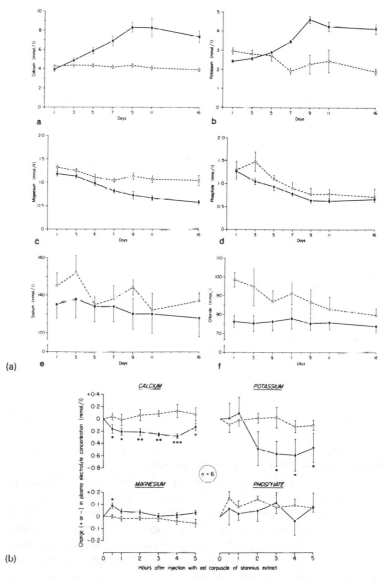

Source: Kenyon, C.J., Chester-Jones, I. and Dixon, R.N.B. (1980) Acute responses of the freshwater eel (*Anguilla anguilla*) to extracts of the corpuscles of Stannius opposing the effects of Stanniosomatiectomy. *Gen. Comp. Endocrinol., 41*, 531-8.

glands are more active in sea water than fresh water. This supports the idea that the corpuscles of Stannius promote hypocalcaemia and removal of the corpuscles of sea water-adapted eels and killifish results in a greater hypercalcaemic response than in fresh water-adapted animals.

Physiology

The hypocalcaemic factor of the corpuscles of Stannius has been named *hypocalcin* but another factor which may or may not be different from hypocalcin has been partially characterised. This factor has been called *teleocalcin* and is a glycopeptide which has been isolated from the corpuscles of Stannius of Pacific salmon. This glycopeptide which has been purified by Sephadex gel filtration, electrophoresis and chromatography has an inhibitory effect on Ca^{2+}-ATPase and is hypocalcaemic in intact American eels. Using this purified glycopeptide it has been shown by studying calcium fluxes across isolated perfused gill systems that hypocalcaemia is probably a result of active branchial calcium uptake mediated by membrane-bound Ca^{2+}-ATPase (Figure 6.3). In those species of teleost with two cell types in the corpuscles it has been shown that the cells are not only structurally different but that they behave differently in experimental situations where the ionic composition of the surrounding water is different and also in salmonids during smoltification and sea-water adaptation. The secretory activity of the type I cell, that is the cells characterised by large electron-dense secretory granules, in three-spined sticklebacks from the sea is much higher than in animals from fresh water. The reverse is true in these fish for the type 2 cells; that is the cells with small secretory granules. If sticklebacks are transferred from sea water to fresh water type 1 cells are inhibited while type 2 cells are stimulated. These changes appear to be similar to those shown by other fish such as the eel and killifish when in sea and fresh water. Even normally fresh water fish when adapted to diluted sea water increase cell size and activity of their type 1 cells. Experiments have clearly shown that it is mainly the calcium concentration of the medium which accounts for the high secretory activity of type 1 cells in sea water. The type 2 cells do not appear to react to variation in calcium content of the ambient medium but probably respond instead to changes in the concentration of sodium and potassium ions in the environment, high concentrations inhibiting their activity. It therefore, seems possible, from morphological studies that the type 2 cells might produce a hormone that stimulates the uptake and/or reduces the losses of sodium and potassium ions. This at the moment cannot be more than a suggestion as sodium/potassium balance in fish is a complicated function involving many hormones and organs.

The coho salmon *Oncorhynchus kisutch* has two types of cells present in the corpuscles of Stannius and these cells both increase in size during smoltification being as large in the freshwater smolts as in the seawater smolts. Also unlike the situation in the three-spined stickleback the type 2 cells in the abnormal stunted salmon in sea water appear to be very active. Why this should be so is not clear. The effect of high calcium concentration on the type 2 cell of the coho salmon is probably a direct one. For isolated Stannius corpuscles have been maintained in organ cultures containing varying concentrations of calcium and the degranulation observed appears related to calcium concentration in the medium. EDTA blocks the effect of high calcium. The response may not, though, be

Figure 6.3: Effects of Extracts of Corpuscles of Stannius on Calcium Influx through the Gill of the Eel. (a) Aqueous extract; (b) partially purified extract.

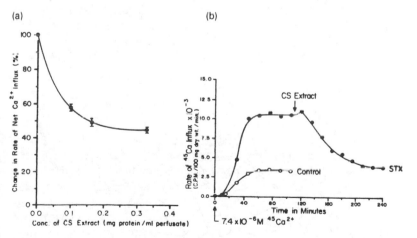

(a)   (b)

Source: Ma, W.Y. and Copp, D.H. (1978) Purification properties and action of a glycopeptide from the corpuscles of Stannius which affect calcium metabolism in the teleost, in P.J. Gaillard and H.H. Böer (eds.) *Comparative Endocrinology*, Elsevier/North Holland, Amsterdam, p. 283.

as direct as it ssems because the presence of nerve fibres and a considerable amount of biogenic amines (noradrenaline, adrenaline and 5-hydroxytryptamine) found in the corpuscles of Stannius suggest that a functional link between neurotransmitters and the type 1 and type 2 cells cannot be excluded (Figure 6.4).

Although it has been suggested that the corpuscles of Stannius produce two factors from distinct cells, the type 1 cell producing the calcium regulating factor and the type 2 cell regulating potassium the proposition in regard to the type 2 cells remains problematic. It has been suggested that the type 2 cells are different physiological stages of the type 1 cells (the immature or post secretory

Figure 6.4: Section through Corpuscles of Stannius Which Shows How 'Adrenergic' Nerve Fibres (AF) Run in the Interlobule Connective Tissue and Approach Both Blood Vessels (B) and Endocrine Cells (EC). These fibres may, in addition to noradrenaline, also store adrenaline and 5-HT. Noradrenaline-storing chromaffin cells (CH) are innervated by cholinergic nerves (CN) and give rise to processes (P)

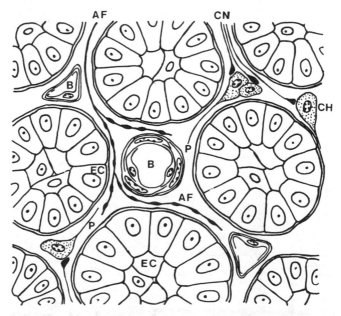

Source: Unsicker, K. *et al.* (1977) Catecholamines and 5-hydroxytryptamine in Corpuscles of Stannius of the salmonid, *Salmo irideus* L. A study correlating electron microscopical, histochemical and chemical findings. *Gen. Comp. Endocrinol., 31*, 121-32.

stages) or that the type 2 cells are also involved in calcium regulation but produce a chemically different hormone. Nevertheless, whether there is one hormone or two or whether or not hypocalcin or teleocalcin are one and the same (they have not been cross tested with their respective assay systems) there is no doubt that calcium homeostasis is a function of the corpuscles of Stannius and possibly the main physiological role of the corpuscles is to maintain the ratio of Ca^{2+} to Na^+ and Cl^- in the plasma.

(b) Urophysis

There occurs in both elasmobranchs and teleosts at the caudal end of the spinal cord a neurosecretory system and a neurohaemal area. This area often forms a very pronounced swelling known as the urophysis (Figure 6.5). In spite of its clear morphological differentiation, its obvious neurosecretory function and its susceptibility to experimental manipulation, only recently has it become established that its products may play a physiological role in osmoregulation.

The morphology of the urophysis was first described in the carp as early as 1827 while the giant caudal neurosecretory neurons were first described in elasmobranchs at the beginning of this century. A well-defined neurohaemal urophysis is seen only in teleost fish. In elasmobranchs the neurosecretory cells, which are called Dahlgren cells and have cell bodies some twenty times larger than ordinary motor neurons, extend along the terminal vertebrae region. The axons of these cells terminate at the blood vessels lying on the latero-ventral surface of the spinal cord. In teleosts the axons of the neurosecretory cells concentrate with blood vessels to form a neurohaemal junction in a manner similar to that seen in the neurohypophysis (Figure 6.6). As with the mammalian neurohypophysis stalk the degree of constriction varies. In some fish such as the eel there is no stalk but only a slight neuro-haemal ventro-lateral swelling of the spinal cord, while in other fish such as *Oryzias*, *Fundulus*, and *Gillichthys* there is a well-defined stalk. In some fish the urophysis is paired, projecting either ventrally or laterally from the cord. The neurosecretory cell bodies lying in the spinal cord have polymorphic nuclei and a basophilic cytoplasm. As the unmyelinated axons of these cells pass into the haemal region to terminate on the capillaries they become enlarged at

Figure 6.5: Section through the Caudal Region of the Spinal Cord
Showing Relation between the Caudal Neurosecretory Neurons
and the Vascular Bed (Cross-hatched) in Four Elasmobranch and
Two Teleost Species.

I   *Squalus acanthias*

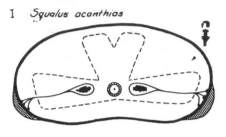

II   *Raia batis*

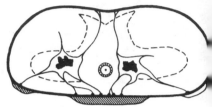

III   *Torpedo ocellata*

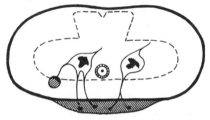

IV   *Trygon violacea*

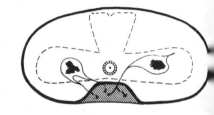

V   *young Esox lucius*

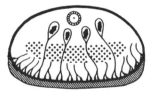

VI   *Leuciscus rutilus*

UROPHYSIS

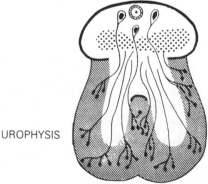

Source: Fridberg, G. (1962). The caudal neurosecretory system in some
elasmobranchs. *Gen. Comp. Endocrinol., 2,* 249-65.

intervals giving rise to Herring bodies. Glial elements and ependymal processes are occasionally seen among the axon terminals as
they discharge their secretion into the basement membranes of the
capillary endothelium.

Although the neurosecretory material of these cells stains well
with certain dyes such as Acid Violet the conventional stains, such

Figure 6.6: Comparison of the Analagous Pattern of Organisation of
the Caudal Secretory System (b) with That of the Hypothalamo-
hypophysial System (a). AH, Adenohypophysis; BV, blood vessels;
CC, central canal; FT, filum terminale; H, Herring body; N, neurohypophysis; P, pituicyte; PV, hypophysial portal vessel; RF,
Reissner's fibre; U, Urophysis.

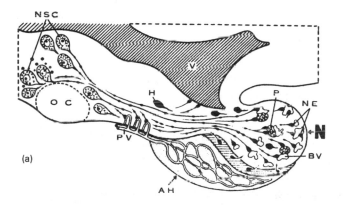

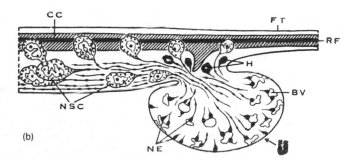

Source: Enami, M. (1958) The morphology and functional significance of the caudal
neurosecretory system of fishes, in A. Gorbman (ed.) *Comparative Endocrinology*, John
Wiley, New York, p 697.

as paraldehyde-fuchsin, chrome-haematoxylin or Alcian blue which are used for the study of the hypothalamic neurosecretory system, do not stain urophysial secretion. The possible intracellular carrier proteins have been termed *urophysins.* There appears to be two or more of these proteins and they are present in elasmobranchs as well as in teleosts. The ultrastructure of the teleost neurosecretory neurons is very similar to that found in all neurosecretory cells with membrane-limited electron-dense granules of 1000-2500 Å (100-250 nm) in diameter in the cell body and 800Å (80 nm) in the region of the end bulbs. In addition to being neurosecretory the neurons possess the electrophysiological properties of neurons, in fact they were the first neurosecretory cells to be shown to have this property. The cells show synaptic transmission and generate spikes characteristic of impulse conduction but their action potential is much longer than that of normal motor neurons. These characteristics apply also to the elasmobranch caudal neurosecretory cells.

Although there is no urophysis as such in elasmobranchs there is a neurohaemal area and a neurosecretory system but no definite neurosecretory cells have been identified in the caudal nerve cord of cyclostomes or holocephalans.

The teleost caudal neurosecretory cell appears to receive a complex neural input. At least two types of aminergic neurons form synapses with the cell body and axon. Electrical stimulation of the urophysial tract leads to discharge or a decreased density of neurosecretory granules.

Following the procedures used to investigate the peptides of the neurohypophysis similar biochemical and pharmacological procedures have isolated a number of peptides in the urophysis. Two biologically active peptides, *urotensin I,* and *urotensin II,* have been well characterised but other active peptides may be produced by the caudal neurosecretory cells. As is conventional in much endocrine investigation acid extracts and acetone powder preparations of both teleost and elasmobranch caudal spinal cord and of the urophysis were tested on various animal tissues. The first thing that was noticed was that these extracts were vasoactive, showing generally a vasopressor response in lower vertebrates and a vasodepressor effect in higher vertebrates. It became evident that these effects were produced by two distinct peptides. These peptides were first separated by Lederis and his colleagues and given the names urotensin I and II. Urotensin I decreases blood pressure in the rat and this decline in blood pressure is caused by vasodilation in skeletal muscle, intestine and visceral organs. However, urotensin I does increase the blood pressure of fish but is very much less potent than urotensin II. This second peptide has a marked effect on blood pressure elevation and also contracts various smooth muscle preparations and increases the urine flow of fish.

Both urotensin I and II appear to be present in all fish so far examined but the presence of two other peptides urotensin III and IV in the urophysis has also been claimed. The presence of a urotensin III is suspected from the fact that urophysial extract injections into goldfish stimulate sodium fluxes across the gill resulting in a net influx whereas urotensin IV appears to be a peptide similar to arginine-vasotocin in that it increases water transfer across the toad urinary bladder.

Although the pharmacology of the urophysial peptides has been critically investigated their chemical properties have not yet been fully determined. Urotensin I has, however, been purified by gel filtration, electrofocusing, ultrafiltration and ion-exchange chromatography. Three fractions of this peptide have been identified with apparently indistinguishable pharmacological properties. The main peptide is a straight chain with about 41 amino acid residues (Figure 6.7). Urotensin II has also been purified and this appears to be a molecule with 23 amino acid residues and two disulphide bridges. Nothing is known of the chemistry of the supposed urotensin III, and urotensin IV, as previously mentioned, which may chemically resemble or indeed be identical with arginine-vasotocin. However, by applying the very sensitive unlabelled antibody peroxidase-antiperoxidase technique to the urophysis of trout no arginine-vasotocin has been demonstrated.

The first experimental studies to determine a possible physiological role for the urophysis were made on the loach, *Misgurnus anguillicaudatus*, in 1956. It was demonstrated that when a single intraperitoneal injection of hypertonic saline was made in this fish there occurred a short increase in secretion from the caudal neurosecretory neuron cell bodies. Repeated injections of salt though caused vacuolisation of these cells and complete loss of secretory activity in the cell bodies. Further evidence that the neurosecretory cells responded to salt levels was obtained by cutting through the spinal cord just anterior to the urophysis. As might be expected the urophysis lost its stainable material but the response

Figure 6.7: Primary Structure of Carp Urotensin I, Sauvagine (Frog Skin Peptide) and Ovine Hypothalamic CRF. Residues underlined are homologous with urotensin I.

```
                                                                              18
UROTENSIN I   H - Asn - Asp - Asp - Pro - Pro - Ile - Ser - Ile - Asp - Leu - Thr - Phe - His - Leu - Leu - Arg - Asn - Met -
                                                                              17
SAUVAGINE       pGlu - Gly - Pro - Pro - Ile - Ser - Ile - Asp - Leu - Ser - Leu - Glu - Leu - Leu - Arg - Lys - Met -
                                                                              18
CRF           H - Ser - Gln - Glu - Pro - Pro - Ile - Ser - Leu - Asp - Leu - Thr - Phe - His - Leu - Leu - Arg - Glu - Val -

                                                                              33
UROTENSIN I   Ile - Glu - Met - Ala - Arg - Asn - Glu - Asn - Gln - Arg - Glu - Gln - Ala - Gly - Leu -
                                                                              32
SAUVAGINE     Ile - Glu - Ile - Glu - Lys - Gln - Glu - Lys - Glu - Lys - Gln - Gln - Ala - Ala - Asn -
                                                                              33
CRF           Leu - Glu - Met - Thr - Lys - Ala - Asp - Gln - Leu - Ala - Gln - Gln - Ala - His - Ser -

                                                                              41
UROTENSIN I   Asn - Arg - Lys - Tyr - Leu - Asp - Glu - Val - NH₂
                                                                              40
SAUVAGINE     Asn - Arg - Leu - Leu - Asp - Thr - Ile - NH₂
                                                                              41
CRF           Asn - Arg - Lys - Leu - Leu - Asp - Ile - Ala - NH₂
```

Source: Ichikawa, T., McMaster, D. and Lederis, K. (1982) Isolation and amino acid sequence of urotensin I, a vasoactive and ACTH-releasing neuropeptide, from the carp (*Cyprinus carpio*) urophysis. *Peptides*, 3, 859-67.

to salt loading of the cell bodies anterior to the cut was a marked increase in the production of neurosecretory material. These results of salt loading on caudal neurosecretion prompted investigations into examining the possibility that the peptides produced by the caudal neurosecretory cells could produce a hormone or hormones concerned directly or indirectly with osmoregulation.

Further experimental evidence provided the information that the incorporation of labelled leucine and tyrosine is much greater in the caudal neurosecretory cells of trout kept in deionised water than those kept in fresh water. Nevertheless the picture remained confused for some years and there was little evidence for the direct action of either urotensin I or urotensin II on ion-transporting cells. The problem was of course that these urophysial peptides could be acting on the vascular system of the gills and kidneys and producing osmoregulatory effects. Recently, however, by using isolated skin preparations free of underlying blood vessels these difficulties have been overcome.

If the isolated skin of the marine teleost *Gillichthys mirabilis* is placed in an Ussing chamber it is found that low concentrations of urotensin I stimulate the short circuit current across the skin and that urotensin I also reverses the inhibition of short-circuit current brought about by adrenaline and urotensin II. As short-circuit current is a measure of active chloride secretion by the marine tele-ost skin (via the chloride secretory cells) then urotensin I and II appear to act on the skin by modulating osmoregulation in at least the marine teleost. The active transport of sodium is also stimu-lated *in vitro* by urotensin II when applied to the urinary bladder of the sea-water acclimated fish *Gillichthys mirabilis*. There is increased transport from the lumen to the serosal side of the bladder and this response is dose related over a physiologically meaningful range of concentrations. Sodium uptake across the intestine of *Ictalurus punctatus* is inhibited by urophysial extracts.

It is now apparent that the involvement of the urophysis in osmoregulation is well established. Lines of evidence from cyto-logical changes of the caudal neurosecretory cells, from alterations in blood ion concentrations, after urophysectomy, from injections of urophysial extracts or urophysins into intact animals and from ion-transport studies on isolated fish tissues, all point to the urophysis playing an important role in salt balance of fish. However, in view of the fact that a number of other hormones in particular cortisol and prolactin are involved in osmoregulation it is still far too early to delineate the exact part played by the urophysins. This will be made easier when it is possible to measure the circulating levels of urophysins in the blood.

Although the urophysis seems mainly concerned with salt balance its products may also play a physiological role in the reproduction of some fish. Urotensin II causes a contraction of the smooth muscle of the urinogenital tract including the sperm duct of *Gillichthys* and also of the oviduct of *Lebistes* suggesting a role for this peptide in oviposition and spawning. Some support for this view is supplied by the fact that the urophysis shows a seasonal change in size in the pike *Esox lucius*. Also depletion of caudal neural granules occurs during the spawning season of *Ompok bimaculatus* and oestrogen treatment causes an enlargement of the caudal neurons while ovariectomy results in a reduction in size of these cells in *Clarias batrachus*. Also the urotensin II content of the sucker, *Catostomus commersoni*, increases towards spawning and falls sharply after spawning.

(c) The Pineal

For many years it was thought that the pineal complex as a dorsal evagination of the brain was a sensory organ in lower vertebrates and a glandular organ in higher vertebrates. Recent research on the pineal in fish, however, has shown that there is a well-defined glandular activity and the current view is that the pineal in cyclostomes and fish, and indeed throughout the vertebrates, is a 'photo-neuroendocrine organ'. Although the gland must now be regarded as the domain of investigation by the endocrinologist the question still persists as to whether the pineal gland of fishes is a vestigial remnant of an ancestral third eye, for numerous investigators have shown that the pineal organ of fishes does have a light receptive function. This function though must, it is thought, have been that of a light 'dosimeter' rather than a true eye for on the top of the head such a structure cannot act as a receptor of a visual field. The modulation of pineal activity by light is probably, in many fish, made via the lateral eyes.

An indole, 5-methoxy-*N*-acetyltryptamine or melatonin, was isolated from the mammalian pineal gland some years ago and has since been shown to be present in all vertebrate classes including fishes. This substance is found only in the pineal and always in very small quantities. It causes a skin lightening reaction when given to amphibians and it is this substance that has been suggested for a physiological role in the pineal related to endocrine function.

Cyclostomes

Development and Structure. In vertebrates two approximately mid-dorsal evaginations develop from the roof of the diencephalon. The more anterior evagination develops into the parapineal body while the pineal organ develops from the more posterior evagination (Figure 6.8). The parapineal is generally absent or rudimentary in adult fish but is well developed in the non-myxinoid cyclostomes. There is very little difference in pineal structure between species in petromyzonts or between the ammocoete and the adult condition. The parapineal tends to lie underneath the pineal. The pineal itself is divided into three main areas; the end bulb, the atrium and the nerve stalk. Pigment cells and sensory cells are found in the lower wall of the end bulb forming the so-called retina. Projections from these sensory cells make contact with 'cones' which project from cells in the roof of the end bulb known as the pellucida. The nerve stalk is made up of cellular elements with very few nerve fibres and connects to the posterior commissure. The three main cell types of the pineal retina, the pigment cells, sensory cells and the ganglion cells are well defined. The parapineal shows no clear demarcation into pellucida and retina, and its lumen is lined by columnar epithelial cells surrounded by a layer of ganglion cells.

Function. The earliest experimental investigation of the possible role of the cyclostome pineal was carried out by J.Z. Young who showed that in the ammocoete larvae of the lamprey removal of the pineal complex caused interruption of the daily rhythm of the integumentary melanophores. These melanophores remained after the operation in an expanded state under all levels of illumination. Thus the normal colour change rhythm shown by ammocoetes, dark by day and pale by night, was abolished leaving the animals permanently dark. It was thought at this time that the paling of the ammocoete when it moved from light to darkness resulted from an inhibition of pituitary melanophore hormone as a result of nervous impulses set up by change of illumination of the pineal complex. More recently in *Lampetra*, and two other species, *Geoteri* and

Figure 6.8: Diagrammatic Sagittal Section through the Pineal of a, a Cyclostome, b, an Elasmobranch, c, a Teleost. HC, commissure, PC, posterior commissure.

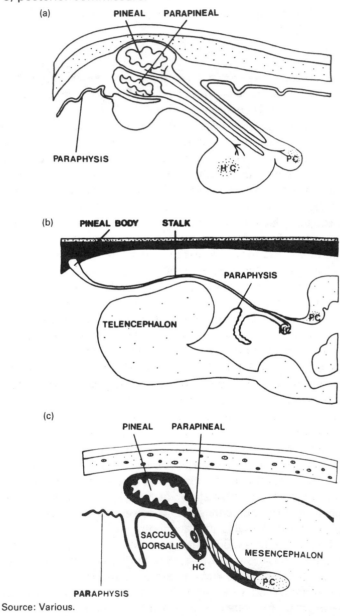

Source: Various.

Mordacia it has now become apparent that the response to light in cyclostomes is both photosensory and endocrinological involving melatonin. Pineal implants into the ammocoetes of *Geoteri* produce an identical melanophore index response to those injected with 5µg melatonin.

Although *Geoteri* ammocoetes like *Lampetra* show a night-time paling and response to melatonin, *Mordacia* displays no night-time paling nor do their melanophores react to melatonin even in very high doses (100µg/animal). Thus there appears to be species differences. Also in these petromyzonts ammocoetes can be made permanently dark by keeping them in continuous light but if they are kept in continuous dark they undergo an increasingly dark to light rhythm until eventually they remain continually dark. It seems then that both pineal and absence of light along with some endogenous factor (perhaps melatonin) are necessary for paling of ammocoetes.

The complexity of colour change in ammocoetes is further demonstrated by the fact that the ammocoetes of *Lampetra* as they grow older diminish the intensity of their diurnal colour change and also by the fact that synthetic melatonin is required in rather large quantities in order to influence the melanophore index of ammocoetes.

Although melatonin itself has not been isolated from the pineal complex of cyclostomes the enzyme hydroxyindole-*O*-methyltransferase (HIOMT) has been identified in the organ. In mammals the enzyme HIOMT is capable of converting *N*-acetyl-serotonin into melatonin and is confined to the pineal and furthermore shows significantly higher activity when associated with dark rather than with light. HIOMT activity has been measured in the pineal complex of *Geotria australis* ammocoetes and found to reach a peak 4 to 5 times that of the basal value between 2 and 3 hours after the onset of darkness (Figure 6.9). This activity is clearly associated with aggregation of pigment in the melanophores. Although melatonin has not been isolated from the cyclostome pineal when [^{3}H]-melatonin is injected it is taken up almost solely by the pineal complex.

Why should certain cyclostome ammocoete larvae show diurnal colour change? What is the usefulness of this to sightless burrowing animals? It has been suggested that the pallor is secondary to the surge of melatonin which is acting as the timer for circadian rhythms of activity within the organs of the ammocoete larvae.

Figure 6.9: HIOMT Activity in the Pineal of Ammocoetes Measured over a 24 Hour Period. The numerals in parentheses are the number of animals contributing to each point. The vertical lines through the means extend 1 standard error of the mean in each direction.

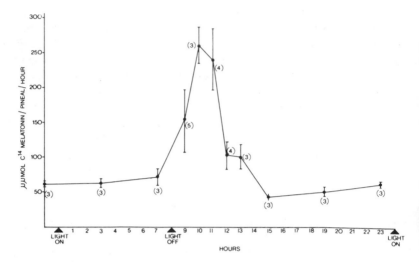

Source: Joss, J.M.P. (1977) Hydroxyindole-*O*-methyltransferase (HIOMT) activity and the uptake of ^{3}H-melatonin in the lamprey, *Geotria australis* Gray. *Gen. Comp. Endocrinol., 31*, 270-5.

This idea is one which suggests that the pineal is a 'biological clock' capable of converting the cyclic nervous activity generated by changes in environmental lighting into endocrine information. The pineal may also convey seasonal information. This last point is borne out by the fact that if the pineal complex is removed from large ammocoetes during a period of six months prior to metamorphosis then these ammocoetes do not metamorphose. Metamorphosis is a phenomenon critically linked to a season.

Osteichthyes

Unlike the situation in the cyclostomes the parapineal in bony fish is either absent or rudimentary. There is, though, a well developed and discrete saccular pineal. Photoreceptors are present which synapse with the afferent nerve tract and many supporting cells are present while the organ is well vascularised. The pineal stalk connects with the subcommissural organ.

When describing the morphology of fish endocrine glands one comes to expect variation in form from species to species. This is so in the case of the pineal of bony fish where the lumen of the vesicular area is much reduced in some species.

The general histological appearance of the fish pineal closely resembles a sensory organ with receptor cells, supporting cells and larger cells with nerve cell characteristics. Although there is a reversed type 'retina' with sensory cells in the inner retinal layer of the distal sac there is no lens-like dorsal pellucida as is seen in cyclostomes. The abundant sensory cells of the organ are large and club-shaped with well-defined nuclei and mitochondria. As in cyclostomes outgrowths from these cells penetrate the lumen of the pineal. The large ganglion or nerve cells are fewer in number. These cells which have a cytology typical of ganglia cells have axons which appear to form the afferent pineal nerve tract. The evidence of there being any efferent fibres originating within the central nervous system and ending on pineal cells is not good.

Recently electron-microscopic studies have been presented which indicate morphological evidence of endocrine activity in the pineal organ of several teleost fish. The sensory cells of *Hyphessobycon scholzei* kept in darkness for several days contain large dense core vesicles of a typical neurosecretory form. Electron dense material is also seen in the intercellular spaces. The support cells may also be active in secretion. In the blind cave-dwelling fish *Typhlichthyes subterraneus* both sensory and supporting cells have well-developed Golgi bodies, clear and dense-cored vesicles, variable amounts of rough endoplasmic reticulum and glycogen particles which indicate that both cell types are metabolically active and possibly play a role in secretion of indoles and/or polypeptides.

Although there is now considerable physiological evidence and some morphological evidence of the pineal of fish functioning as an endocrine gland there is little doubt that the pineal complex of most fish functions as a sensory organ. That the pineal in fish may be receptive to light intensity is borne out by the fact that bony fish can be divided into three groups with respect to the organisation of the tissues that cover the pineal organ. In one group of fish the tissue overlying the pineal is transparent and forms a 'pineal window'. In a second group entrance of light into the pineal appears to be regulated by appropriately placed chromatophores while in a third group the tissues over the pineal are opaque.

Species with a 'pineal window' show positive phototactic movement while those with an opaque pineal covering show negative
phototactic movements. The role of the pineal body as a sensory
organ in fish has been reviewed by a number of authors and
therefore only the endocrine function of the gland will now be discussed.

The pineal gland of bony fish contains melatonin, the enzyme
HIOMT necessary for the formation of melatonin, serotonin and a
number of free amino acids which may all act as chemical trans-
mitters and have some physiological role. The gland appears to
have a high metabolic rate and takes up radioactive phosphorus
more rapidly than any other tissue in the fish body. The enzyme
HIOMT has been characterised in the juvenile chinook salmon,
Oncorhynchus tschawytscha. It has also been found in the retina and
the dorsal portion of the diencephalon but in much smaller
amounts than in the pineal.

Melatonin, serotonin and HIOMT have all been estimated
quantitatively in the pineal and plasma of bony fish. Plasma mela-

Figure 6.10: Plasma Melatonin in Trout ($n = 8$) during the Day and
Night. Night levels were significantly ($P < 0.01$) elevated over the
photophase levels, as tested by paired-comparison analysis of
variance.

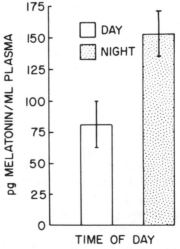

Source: Gern, W.A., Owens, D.W. and Ralph, C.L. (1978) Plasma melatonin in the trout:
day-night change demonstrated by radioimmunoassay. *Gen. Comp. Endocrinol., 34,*
453-8.

Figure 6.11: Diurnal Variation of 5-HT Content in the Pineal Organ of the Yellow Eel. Dark fields represent dark phase of light regime (LD 12:12).

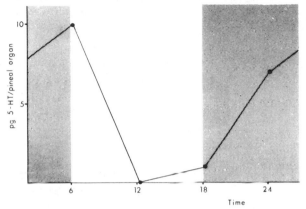

Source: van Veen, T., Laxmyr, L. and Borg, B. (1982) Diurnal variation of 5-hydroxytryptamine content in the pineal organ of the yellow eel (*Anguilla anguilla* (L)). *Gen. Comp. Endocrinol.*, *46*, 322-6.

tonin when measured by radioimmunoassay in the rainbow trout shows a marked daily rhythm (Figure 6.10) as does serotonin content of the yellow eel pineal (Figure 6.11). While it was initially thought that HIOMT levels in the pineal showed a diurnal rhythm it has been more recently shown that the variation in specific activity is related to changes in the protein content of the gland.

Do changes in melatonin in the plasma influence release of pituitary or other hormones or do they directly effect the biochemistry of fish? Injection of melatonin or pineal extracts and pinealectomy have all been performed in an endeavour to answer this question.

If teleosts are injected with, or immersed in, a solution of melatonin generally there is a lightening of the skin caused by contraction of melanophores. Sometimes, however, melatonin can act as a darkening agent. In the pencil fish *Nammostomus beckfordi anomalus* which has separate day and night markings the addition of melatonin to the water produces a night coloration within 5-15 minutes at concentrations as low as 0.03μg/ml. The melatonin causes the melanophores of the night spots to expand and the day band to contract. The melatonin induced night colours remain for periods of up to one hour before the day-band starts to reappear. This provides some indirect evidence for the involvement of melatonin in the control of circadian pigment rhythms in teleosts.

The removal of the pineal has been carried out in a number of teleost species both to investigate the gland's effect on skin pigmentation and on other possible roles. Results though have been somewhat equivocal. This is possibly due to the fact that in some species of fish the anterior brain region appears to be photoreceptive in itself, and this makes the interpretation of such experiments difficult and the effect of pineal removal often seems to have been dependent on the involvement of the neighbouring brain regions. Also the time of year at which pinealectomy is performed seems to influence the results obtained. It must be remembered that there is in teleost fish a variation from entirely neural to predominantly hormonal control of melanophores. Neural control is seen in the minnow, *Phoxinus phoxinus,* the guppy and the killifish while hormonal control is evident in the eel. Neural control of melanophore pigment aggregation and dispersion in teleosts is primarily mediated through sympathetic innervation. Although melatonin has no effect on the melanophores of killifish if this animal is pinealectomised there is elimination of the circadian rhythm of colour change but no effect on physiological colour change and background adaptation. The pinealectomy of other teleosts disturbs their circadian organisation and rhythmicity.

This effect of pinealectomy on physiological rhythms of fish is now well established. Pinealectomy of the goldfish abolishes its liver glycogen daily variation, modifies plasma glucose variation and lipid rhythms are also altered. Growth and plasma mineral levels may also be modified by pinealectomy but these modifications seem always related to time of day or season of the year. It may be then that melatonin is a pineal hormone whose function is to transduce or mediate photoperiod information by modifying hypothalamic — pituitary function and hence metabolic processes in fish.

This possible role may be extended into a relationship with reproduction. The pineal/gonadal relationship is well known in mammals although the precise and particular mechanism and action of the pineal in reproduction is not obvious. In a number of higher vertebrates the most important function of the pineal appears to be its ability to control or modulate seasonal reproductive rhythms. In, for example, the hamster, under short photoperiods either in the laboratory or under reducing natural day length the gonads become completely degenerated but pinealectomy prevents this dark-induced gonadal involution. Thus the pineal hormone appears to suppress the reproductive state. In the fish, *Fundulus*, melatonin, depending on the period of the year at which it is administered, effects gonad development. Melatonin-treated fish collected in January or May and maintained in long photoperiods have significantly smaller gonads than control animals. Also melatonin treatment of male fish maintained on a short photoperiod in May retarded testis enlargement but similar treatment on animals kept on a short photoperiod in January had no effect. Gonadal size in goldfish is also seasonally pineal dependent. If bull pineal extract is fed to *Poecilia reticulata* the appearance of secondary sexual characteristics is delayed while in the same species pinealectomy accelerates sexual maturation. The exact role of melatonin in gonadal inhibition of fish is unknown but the pineal in fish acts in some way as a dosimeter and trans-ducer of radiation effecting reproductive and pigmentary responses. There is, however, an indication that gonadotropin secretion is affected by the pineal. Pinealectomy of goldfish represses the daily cycle of plasma gonadotropin. In spring the pineal seems to stimulate gonadal development by promoting a daily cycle in serum gonadotropin levels under long photoperiod and to suppress gonadal development by inhibiting the cycle under short photoperiod.

Melatonin has been found to decrease the locomotor activity that occurs during the light phase of the fish photoperiod; on the other hand serotonin increases locomotor activity during the dark period. In spite of these suggestive observations the role of the pineal, if any, in the control of the locomotor behaviour of fish has yet to be established.

Chondrichthyes

Very little is known about the pineal of elasmobranchs. A photo-receptor capacity has been demonstrated for the pineal of the dog-fish, *Scyliorhinus canicula.* The spontaneous activity of the pineal nerve fibres is influenced by light and the duration of this inhibi-tion is proportional to light intensity. In the absence of light morphological changes occur in various pineal cells, however, con-tinuous illumination produces no structural effects within the cells. No diurnal changes have been observed in the histology of the cells. The effects of removal of the pineal gland have not been studied in any elasmobranch neither has the presence of melatonin in the gland been detected.

7 PHEROMONES

Chemical signals carrying information from one animal to another are common in the animal kingdom. The fox-hound sniffing out the fox, the female cat attracting the male, the pungent odour of the skunk when cornered are all examples of chemical interactions between animals. Such chemical substances in general are called *semiochemicals* and they can interact between individuals of different species in which case they are known as *allomones* (interspecific semiochemicals) or the interaction can be between individuals of the same species in which case they are known as *pheromones* (intraspecific semiochemicals).

Chemical signalling systems are found in many phyla and involve many different chemicals. The reception of these signals takes place either by olfaction or gustation (tasting). The allomones and pheromones of fish are secretions released into the external medium, water, conveying information usually via olfactory receptors and bringing about fairly specific reactions and behavioural changes in the recipient. Allomones have been defined as chemical agents of adaptive value to the organism producing them and not acting between members of the same species. Allomones may be chemicals secreted for attack (venoms) or defence (the formic acid of ants). Pheromones, however, act in minute amounts within a defined context and between individuals of a single species. They are either *releasers*, which trigger a relatively rapid behaviour response, or *primers*, which usually involve the endocrine system and produce a more gradual and prolonged shift in the physiology of the recipient. In a discussion of fish endocrinology when the main theme is an account of chemical messengers transmitted internally and which evoke responses in the individuals secreting them, it seems perfectly reasonable to extend this concept to chemicals which are transmitted externally between animals of the same species. The isolation of pheromones and knowledge of their activity now forms a part of the science of endocrinology for as has been already said both internal specific secretions and external secretion are but two bands of the spectrum of chemical communication. Accordingly the role of pheromones in fish will be described here but not that of allomones.

198

The pheromones of fish may be described under three main headings, alarm and social behaviour substances, species and sex recognition and sex behavioural inducing substances, and finally territorial and space recognition substances.

Like other invertebrates and vertebrates fish rely on a complex multisensory communication system for their social and sexual interactions. Chemoreception although not as fast as visual or auditory perception is extremely sensitive and was possibly developed early in evolution. However, whereas in invertebrates pheromones have developed to induce a stereotyped behavioural or developmental response in the recipient organism in fish, as in other vertebrates, this response is much more varied.

Alarm and Social Behaviour Pheromones

Alarm substances have been demonstrated to occur in the skin of certain fish such as the minnow, *Phoxinus phoxinus*. The pheromone appears to be stored in specialised epidermal cells, the club cells, which release the pheromone only when the cell is broken by a mechanical injury to the skin. The pheromone causes the fish to scatter and particularly if a predator in the process of eating a minnow releases the substance other fish are helped to escape further attack. Surprisingly, however, the active pheromone does hardly appear to be released at all in the case of cannibalism. The alarm substance also appears to be reduced in the skins of spawning male and female minnows, and also in starved or unhealthy individuals. Perhaps there is an adaptive value here.

The chemical nature of alarm substances is not known but they are apparently heat-labile and water-soluble and it has been suggested that they may be pterines or aminosugars. The alarm substance is not present in many groups of fish, particularly in shoaling fish, e.g. clupidae and percidae. Also the ability both to respond to and to produce alarm substances is not present on hatching. It takes about a month for the substance to appear in minnows and, in common with conventional hormone action, pheromones such as alarm substances act in very low concentrations. Extracts made from a 200 mg lacerated piece of minnow skin can be detected by minnows at a dilution of 1 in 50,000.

Chemical communication also appears to direct other social behavioural aspects of fish in addition to the alarm or fright

reaction. For example hierarchical behaviour and schooling are influenced by pheromones. Probably the best-known example of social
hierarchy and pheromone influence is seen in the yellow bullhead,
Ictalurus natalis. Individuals of this species can be trained by
operant conditioning techniques (reward/punishment) to discriminate between the smell of two other fish of the same species.
Utilising this phenomenon and knowing the behavioural pattern
shown by these fish when dominance is disputed it has been shown
that water from a tank holding a previously established dominant
initiated submissive behaviour. Also it has been found that water
from a tank holding submissives caused dominants to attack.
Another interesting feature in this animal is that chemical recognition of dominance of an individual disappeared after it had been
defeated in an encounter. Nothing is known of the chemicals that
produce these behavioural patterns but it seems that there is more
than one.

The catfish, *Ictalurus nebulosus*, provides cues for individual
recognition by urine and not by mucous secretion as probably does
the yellow bullhead. It has been suggested that this pheromone in
the urine is derived from the urohypophysis.

The schooling behaviour seen in many species of fish is largely
visual during the day but does appear to be controlled by
olfaction particularly at night. Blind rudd fail to maintain a proper
school but do remain in the area of odour of other rudd. The
minnow, *Phoxinus phoxinus*, maintain schools because of odours
released from the skin mucus and in the catfish eel, *Plotosus
anguillaris*, this schooling substance has been shown to be dialys-
able and heat stable.

Sex Recognition and Behaviour

Fish, and here we refer to teleosts, for little or no information is
available on cyclostomes and elasmobranchs, have exploited
chemical communication for both the control of fertility and the
co-ordination of sexual and epigamic behaviours. Control of fertility as will be mentioned later may be regarded as part of the
pheromonal relation to crowding. Male guppies are attracted by
the odour of female guppies as are male *Ictalurus punctatus* and
Brachydanio rerio. In a number of other fish, however, including
the rainbow trout the male is only attracted by the odour of the

ovulated or ripe female. In some species males are induced to interact more vigorously by female odours while in other species it is the male odour that attracts females. Thus, there appears to be many permutations and combinations of sexual attractants in teleosts. Unfortunately, once more virtually nothing is known of their chemical composition. Sex steroids may be involved because a change in the electrical activity of the olfactory bulbs, both evoked and spontaneous, has been reported in male goldfish treated with sex hormones. Also ripe male goldfish are able to discriminate between ovulated and unovulated females by a pheromone contained in the ovarian fluid which is released shortly after ovulation. A number of other species such as gobies and loach contain ovarian pheromones which elicit courtship. A testicular sex pheromone has been postulated to occur in the black goby.

Attractant substances derived from the gonads may not be the only source of sex pheromones for the holding water of adult virgin female guppies, *Poecilia reticulata*, whose oviduct is closed still attracts males. It is most probable though that an ovarian pheromone generally is released into the urine and hence to the exterior. However, owing to peripheral metabolism and binding to plasma proteins it is not likely that an ovarian steroid hormone itself acts as the urinary pheromone. Male guppies are attracted to water which has previously held females but *not* to control water or water in which males or ovariectomised females have been maintained. Also they express preference for the kind of water. The males prefer water which has held females for the first few days of their gestation cycle over water which has held gravid females. Male courtship is induced when water which has held an intact female is added to water containing an ovariectomised female.

Similar demonstrations have been made in a number of teleosts of female sex pheromones produced by the ovary of the female, serving to synchronise maximum sexual activity and increasing the likelihood of insemination with the time of maturation of the ova.

It is unlikely, as previously mentioned, that teleost female sex pheromones are oestrogens in spite of the fact that steroids can evoke olfactory bulb potentials. A number of different chemicals have been proposed. In the rainbow trout both water-soluble and an ether-soluble basic component have been identified; in the goldfish an ether-soluble substance; in *Hypomesus oliduse*, a protein and in *Brachydanio rerio*, a steroid glucuronide. At present a very likely candidate or candidates for a sex pheromone in fish appears to be steroid glucuronides. Both male goldfish and guppies are attracted by aetiocholanolone glucuronide whereas females do not react.

Territory and Space Recognition

Pheromones appear to play an important part in the recognition and the response to environment in teleosts. Many species of fish are capable of conditioning the surrounding water to produce an effect on other individuals. The chemical cues thus produced facilitate or inhibit growth or control fertility. The 'conditioning' of water so that fish live better in water where other fish have lived has been known by tropical aquarium fish keepers for many years. Goldfish show a significant increase in their growth rate when reared in water (filtered to remove the food particles) which has previously contained goldfish. The conditioning or growth promoting substance appears to be contained in the epidermal mucus. Rainbow trout respond better to stress in 'conditioned' water. If the water in which trout are subject to thermal stress until heat death is used to thermal stress a second batch of trout then this second batch take longer for heat death to occur. The water has been 'conditioned'.

More common than the beneficial effects on fish found in 'conditioned' water are the inhibiting effects produced on growth and particularly the inhibiting growth factors produced by crowding. The decrease in growth rate or stunting brought about by crowded conditions has been recognised for a long time. However, it was not until 1959 that Rose examined several species of fish under densely crowded conditions. His first experiments were with the white cloud mountain fish, *Tanichthys albonubes*. He found that in a 15 litre aquarium a breeding pair of fish produces up to 200 fertile eggs but only 20 fish grow to 1 cm in length. Another fish, *Barbus tetrazona*, was similar in its growth and development pattern. Size differences became apparent shortly after feeding commenced in both species of fish. Larger fish continued to grow but smaller fish stopped eating and died. These smaller fish if they were removed to another tank grew well. In *Barbus tetrazona* also only 15 1 cm fish survived from 200 eggs but if the water in the tank was changed daily about 170 fish survived to 1 cm. This demonstrated that the effect was not a physical one.

The growth-inhibiting factor of *Brachydanio rerio* has been extracted and it appears to be a lipoidal chloroform extractable substance. Inhibitors other than those affecting growth appear to be present in fish. Crowding has been shown to promote the release of a heart-rate depressant in goldfish and of an immuno-suppressive factor in the blue gourami, *Trichogaster tricopterus.*

It has been suggested that the main function of crowding factors is in fact to prevent crowding by favouring fish dispersal. Although the relationship of pheromones to schooling has already been mentioned, there is what can be considered as a specialised type of schooling or aggregating behaviour, namely *the homing behaviour* of migrating fish. Although migration and the role of hormones in the phenomenon will be discussed in Chapter 8 in detail of homeward migration of fish can well be discussed here in the context of pheromone production.

It was suggested many years ago that the Atlantic salmon, *Salmo salar,* responded to odours produced by the young fish in the river but it was thought rather unlikely. Some experimental evidence became available when of two branches of the Apple river in Nova Scotia salmon were found to ascend only the west branch although there was no barrier to prevent them ascending the east branch where a mill dam had been removed some ten years earlier. This was in 1932. However, in that year fry were planted in the east branch and later that year there was a considerable run of adults into this stream. It seemed that the presence of young fish in the stream had made it attractive to adult fish. More recently it was suggested that a race-specific odour from young migratory char, *Salvelinus alpinus,* attracts adults of that race. This was established by taking artificially fertilised eggs, rearing them several hundred kilometres from their river of origin for four years, releasing them and finding that two-thirds of those released returned to the river which was known only to their parents and relatives. It was concluded that a race-specific odour emanated from the river. Other experiments with tagged char have confirmed this homing to relatives occupying a restricted portion of the river.

The anadromous migratory char is also a very good fish for this type of experiment because it takes to sea once every summer during the post-smolt stage and always returns to its respective fresh water locality. Other salmon also perform remarkable and well-timed migration from feeding areas at sea to their home river but generally spend a longer time at sea than char. The seasonal homeward migration of both Pacific and Atlantic salmon is divided into (a) the timing of the start of the homeward migration, (b) the choice of migratory direction and the maintenance of course in open sea and coastal waters and (c) the selection of home river and localisation of the area of origin in that river system. The analysis and the understanding of the physiology, behaviour and the nature of environmental and biological cues in all these stages of homeward migration of salmonids is complex; only (c) will be discussed here.

The artificial orientation of homeward migration and river selection is now thought to depend upon the recognition of characteristic water odours of the freshwater home areas imprinted before sea-water migration as smolt. The possibility that fish are guided to their home stream by non-pheromonal chemical cues must always be borne in mind. These can even come from the soil or from plants and are encountered and can be imprinted during smoltification. However, there is similar evidence to support the pheromone hypothesis of homing from the Atlantic salmon in addition to that from char.

In addition to field observations made with transplanted stock of salmonids laboratory experiments of recordings from single cells in the olfactory bulb of the char have been made. These show that fish can discriminate char populations from different areas on the basis of odorants contained in the epidermal mucus. The slime secreted by fish is generous and could well supply the chemical basis for an olfactory attractant. Furthermore, differential responses of the olfactory bulbs have been observed to homo- and heterospecific skin mucus in the rainbow trout.

Not only salmonids may release a homing pheromone but it is of interest that elvers of the catadromous species, *Anguilla rostrata*, are drawn upstream by a heat-stable non-volatile substance produced by the adult eel and not by the young as in salmonids.

The chemical fractionation of the skin mucus and an isolation of a homing pheromone has not proved easy. Contamination of samples with urine or faeces is always a possibility. Certain low molecular weight substances from home stream water act as olfactory stimulants to alewives, *Alosa pseudoharangus*, whereas bile salts have been implicated as probable homing pheromones in char.

8 HORMONES, MIGRATION AND SEA-RANCHING

Migration

The phenomenon of animal migration has attracted biologists of many kinds, ecologists, physiologists, behaviourists, neurophysiologists and many others including endocrinologists. Many species of fish are migratory including some of great commercial importance and it is, therefore, not surprising that much fish endocrinology has been directed towards this phenomenon. Migration in fish is generally regarded, as in other animals, as an adaptive strategy for increasing growth, survival and abundance. It has been argued that abundance results in commercial interest and this would explain why important commercial species are migratory. This is however, a matter for discussion.

Fish migration has been well reviewed by many including Hasler (1966), Harden Jones (1968), Northcote (1978) and McKeown (1984). All tend to classify migratory movements into 'micro-migrations' occurring over short periods of time and 'macro-migrations'. It is these large-scale migrations that have concerned the physiologist and endocrinologists particularly when movement from fresh water to salt water or vice-versa occurs with subsequent osmoregulatory changes. However, it must be remembered that these are the regulatory changes that must take place if the fish is to optimise the utilisation of the most favourable resources and habitat during the feeding or reproductive phases of its life history.

The cyclostomes migrate. Although the myxinoids are exclusively marine and show little if any 'micro-migration' the petromyzonts are often amphihaline, that is they migrate between fresh water and sea water. In the metamorphosis of the ammocoete larva of the river lamprey, *Lampetra fluviatilis*, endocrinological changes take place in the pancreas, the adrenal tissue and most obviously in the transformation of the endostyle into the adult thyroid gland. However, these changes must be regarded as developmental rather than specifically related to the phenomenon of migration. In cyclostomes no endocrine factor has been identified either as a causative agent in the initiation of either downstream or upstream migrations or as a necessary factor in the maintenance of the homeostatic state of the animal when undergoing salinity transference.

Teleost fish may be amphihaline (migration between salt and fresh water), holohaline (migration in water of the same salinity), catadromous (a downstream migrant) or anadromous (an upstream migrant). Also species may be classified as amphihaline potamotocous when they reproduce in fresh water as in the case of salmon and amphihaline thalassotocous when they reproduce in sea water as do the eels. Very few endocrine investigations have been made upon holohaline fish and these will be mentioned later. The vast amount of information that we have concerns amphihaline potamotocous or thalassotocous fish, and this is restricted largely to the eel, the Atlantic salmon and the Pacific salmon. The metabolic changes related to spawning migration of these animals are great; the accumulation of sufficient energy reserves to withstand long periods of nonfeeding; the stress responses required to cope with changed environments and osmotic mileu; the demands of sexual behaviour and spawning, all bring into play hormones. Do these hormones act only as regulators or modulators of the homeostatic state of the fish and controllers of the reproductive process or is the phenomenon of migration a response to endocrine change? No answer is yet available.

The Atlantic salmon, *Salmo salar*, enters the rivers at all times of the year returning to freshwater as a 'salmon' (after 2-4 years at sea) or a 'grilse' (after 1 year + at sea). Proceeding up river the fish do not feed. Egg laying starts in the late autumn and they hatch in March as alevins. These larvae grow into parr which live in the upland streams for one to four years. Metamorphosis from parr to smolt takes place when the fish turn silver and change body shape. At this stage the smolt migrates to the sea, but not necessarily all at the same time (nor do they return at the same time). This variability of upstream and downstream migration obviously has survival value for the species. This brief description of the Atlantic salmon life history makes it evident that endocrine regulation is involved. The Pacific salmon of the genus *Oncorhynchus* show similar life histories but as there are five migratory species and several land-locked species there is variation. For example *Oncorhynchus keta*, the chum salmon, and *O. gorbuscha*, the pink salmon, are born near the sea and assume an oceanic life soon after hatching. In these species there is a suppression or loss of the parr stage.

The thyroid gland was perhaps the first endocrine gland to be implicated in migratory processes. This occurred when over forty years ago Hoar pointed out an active hyperplasia of the thyroid gland during the smolt stage of salmon and Landgrebe demonstrated that thyroid hormones induced the appearance of silvering in parr. This gave rise to the view that smoltification might be directly dependent upon the thyroid. An increase in thyroid hormone secretion was found during the parr-smolt transformation. However, thyroid feeding was unable to prevent the depression of the hypo-osmotic regulation capacity of smolt during the desmoltification and radiothyroidectomy did not inhibit smolt transformation and migration. Nevertheless thyroxine and anti-thyroid drugs influence the salinity preferences of young salmon. Also changes in swimming activity can be induced by thyroid hormones during the parr smolt transformation and it has been suggested that a normal physiological role in thyroid activity would increase motor activity required for seaward migration.

Some experiments have shown that trout 'smoltified' by thyroid hormone treatment increase euryhalinity and this is held to be evidence for a similar process existing in salmon. As thyroid hormone activity in fish is related to growth (Chapter 2) a reduction in thyroid hormone production which occurs after sea-water entry in the coho salmon has been related to growth cessation. Also the peaks and seasonal cycles of thyroid hormone production which are seen in fresh-water salmonids and which have been correlated with gonadal development have also been seen in migratory salmonids but here they appear to coincide with the period of smoltification. This last observation has raised considerable interest over the past few years.

Plasma thyroxine was first measured in coho salmon during the smoltification process through the early spring and showed a distinct peak (Figure 8.1). At this point the significance of this surge was not known but was confirmed on the masu salmon, *Oncorhynchus masou*, of Japan where a peak of thyroxine occurred during April when parr-smolt transformation was proceeding (Figure 8.2). An advance was made when it was discovered that the lunar cycle plays an important part in the temporal organisation of smoltification. An analysis by Grau and his colleagues in 1981 of 27 groups of hatchery-reared coho salmon and anadromous trout indicated that the peak thyroxine levels occurred at the period of the new moon (Figure 8.3). The outward migration of

Figure 8.1: Plasma Thyroxine Concentrations during Smoltification of Coho Salmon from Big Creek (●) and Kalama (Δ) Hatcheries. Each symbol represents mean of 10 plasma samples; brackets include ± SE.

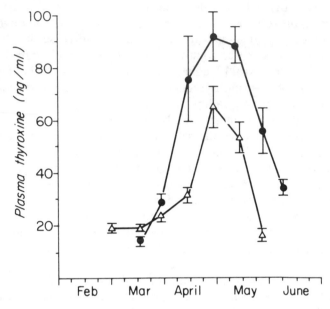

Source: Dickhoff, W.W., Folmar, L.C. and Gorbman, A. (1978) Changes in plasma thyroxine during smoltification of coho salmon, *Oncorhynchus kisutch. Gen. Comp. Endocrinol., 36*, 229-32.

coho salmon is known to peak at the full moon. Perhaps this migration is related to the surge of thyroxine influencing growth, migratory restlessness and sea water preference prior to the full moon. This is possibly the optimum method of synchrony to ensure an efficient and sequentially well-ordered role for the thyroid in its relation to the migratory process. There appears little doubt now that in coho and perhaps chinook salmon the plasma surge of thyroxine and the lunar cycle are a 'phase locked' smoltification-related phenomenon.

It is well known that gill sodium-potassium activated adenosine triphosphatase (Na^+,K^+-ATPase) is an important component of osmoregulation in sea water. The activity of this enzyme has been observed to increase in migrating smolts prior to sea water entry. However, the exact mechanism by which environmental changes

Figure 8.2: Seasonal Changes in the Serum Levels of Thyroxine (T_4) and Triiodothyronine (T_3) in Masu Salmon. Each point indicates the concentration of T_4 and T_3 in the serum, in female smolt (●), male smolt (▲), female parr (○) and male parr (△). A solid line indicates the mean of smolt, and a broken line indicates the mean of parr. In some specimens, T_4 was not detectable. These specimens were regarded as 0 μg when the average was calculated.

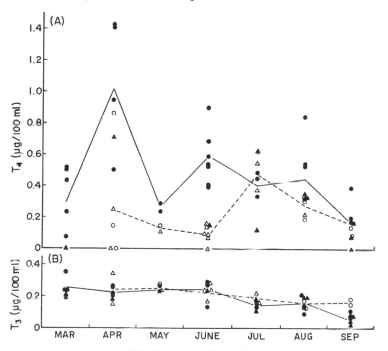

Source: Nishikawa, K. *et al.* (1979) Changes in circulating L-thyroxine and L-triiodothyronine of the masu salmon, *Oncorhynchus masou* accompanying the smoltification, measured by radioimmunoassay. *Endocrinol. Japan, 26(6)*, 731-5.

stimulate Na^+,K^+-ATPase is unknown but a number of hormones including thyroxine have been implicated. There is some evidence of thyroxine changes in the plasma being correlated with the increase in Na^+,K^+-ATPase which occurs during the acclimation of coho salmon smolts to sea water but this does no more than perhaps suggest a causal relationship. In fact some experiments have not been able to establish any consistent change in plasma thyroid hormone levels when coho salmon are transferred to sea water.

Figure 8.3: Patterns of Plasma T_4 in Three California Coho Salmon Stocks Plotted on a Lunar Calendar. ●, new moon; ○, full moon.

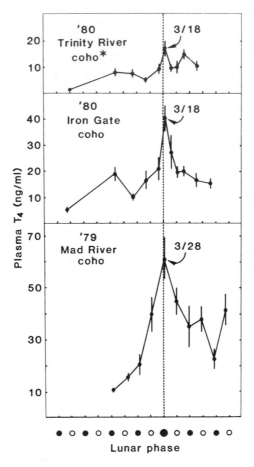

Source: Grau, E.G. *et al*. (1981) Lunar phasing of the thyroxine surge preparatory to seaward migration of salmonid fish. *Science, 211*, 607-9.

In addition to changes taking place in thyroid hormone levels of salmon undergoing parr-smolt transformation, and in seaward migration, thyroxine levels change during the upstream reproductive migration. The changes are more marked in the male than in the female salmon. There is, both in the Atlantic and the Pacific salmon, a general decrease in thyroid activity as the fish, both the male and female, migrate upstream in fresh water until they spawn.

Changes in thyroid activity take place during the various migratory and metamorphic changes that take place during the life history of the eel. Many of the changes have been observed histologically which is a very indirect and uncertain method of assessing endocrine gland activity. (Does a highly vacuolated and high columnar celled thyroid follicles mean high hormone activity or a phase of hormone production exhaustion?) There is, though, increased activity of the thyroid during the transformation of the yellow eel into the silver eel. European silver eels during the autumn make efforts to leave the water environment and often in the wild one finds in the morning eels making their way across damp fields. With analogy to the tadpole-frog metamorphosis and amphibian terrestrial development being related to thyroid activity, in the past a number of investigators have related terrestrial phases in fish to increased thyroid activity. In fact many years ago it was claimed that thyroid hormone treatment caused gobies and blennies to become terrestrial (rather like the amphibious Periophthalmids). This observation has not been confirmed. Also examination of the thyroids of the leptocephalus larvae as they metamorphose into elvers indicates an active gland. The thyroid gland may play a role in the migratory mechanism of holohaline fish. Histological observations on the cod *Gadus callarias* have shown both in adult and immature fish a cycle of activity in the thyroid beginning at the start of its southward migration over the Bear Island-Spitsbergen Bank and ending when the fish reach their spawning grounds off the Lofoten Islands. The thyroid of sardine and tuna have been studied during their movements in the sea and thyroid activity variations noted. It is difficult, though, to conclude anything definite about the gland and migration from these observations.

Perhaps some of the most suggestive experiments linking the thyroid gland with the migratory process have been those of Bertha Baggerman. In a series of studies she examined changes in salinity preference shown by salmon and sticklebacks after hormone treatment. Fish were placed in a trough in which one half contained salt water and the other half fresh water separated by a glass partition. Both compartments were connected by a layer of fresh water which was allowed to flow over the partition. Fish were thus enabled to swim freely from one compartment to the other. By this means salinity preference could be established and analysed. Sticklebacks show a strong fresh-water preference after treatment with thyroxine or TSH (Figure 8.4) whereas Pacific salmon show a strong salt-water preference after TSH injection (Figure 8.5). Baggerman further established that in yearling coho salmon a long daylength given in the early months of the year promoted the onset of the change in salinity preference. This suggested that the change in salinity preference which occurs at the onset of seaward migration is mainly brought about by the long spring days and make it very likely that the endocrine system is involved by the way of the hypothalamo-pituitary axis.

Another gland that has been implicated in the phenomenon of fish migration is the interrenal. As seen in Chapter 4 osmoregulation by teleosts in seawater appears to be influenced by cortisol even though the exact physiological role of the hormone is uncertain. Also cortisol has been shown to increase Na^+ excretion, water permeability and Na^+,K^+-ATPase activity of the gill along with water and ion movement in the intestine and urinary bladder. Activation of the pituitary-interrenal axis has been observed in smolting salmon but little is really known of the physiological role of cortisol in smoltification or sea-water adaptation. Elevated blood corticosteroids occur in salmonids during sexual maturation and it has been suggested that corticosteroids are responsible for induction of oocyte maturation, for coping with the stress of salt water-fresh water change, and for the gluconeogenesis required of non-feeding animals. In the case of Pacific salmon the stress response apparently cannot be met, the interrenals become exhausted and death of all fish occurs after spawning. Atlantic salmon are more successful and a number return to the sea after spawning.

Corticosteroid levels vary in the plasma of eels during their life cycle and appear to influence hydro-mineral metabolism. Having said this one can say little more about the normal physiological changes in these hormones taking place during migration. Certainly the interrenals must take some part in the stresses of migration and in the gluconeogenesis needed by the fasting silver eel as it swims downstream.

It would be surprising if the pituitary played no role in migration. Certainly thyroidal changes and changes in plasma corticosteroid levels during different migratory phases must be modulated by TSH or ACTH. For many years morphological and cytological changes have been reported in salmon and eel pituitaries. The degranulation of the pituitary thyrotrophs suggests a release of TSH

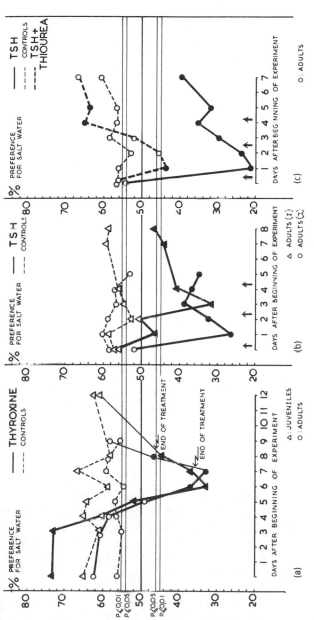

Figure 8.4: Stickleback (*Gasterosteus aculeatus*) Salinity Preference. Changes in salinity preference induced by treatment with a: thyroxine, b: TSH + thiourea and c: TSH. Solid symbols represent a significant difference (*P* = ≤ 0.05) between the treated groups and their controls. Arrows indicate days on which injections were given. For further information see text.

Source: Baggerman, B. (1962) Some endocrine aspects of fish migration. *Gen. Comp. Endocrinol., Suppl. 1*, 188-205.

Figure 8.5: Average Percentage Preference for Saltwater in Coho Juveniles after Treatment with TSH (0.05 I.U./Injection). Vertical lines represent the extremes in preference as shown by the different groups. Horizontal drawn and broken lines indicate levels at which the preference for salt- (or fresh-water) are significant to the 0.05 and 0.01 levels.

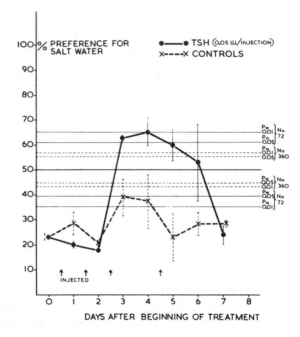

Source: Baggerman, B. (1963) The effect of TSH and antithyroid substances on salinity preference and thyroid activity in juvenile Pacific salmon. *Can. J. Zool., 41*, 307-19.

which is responsible for the stimulation of the thyroid which modifies a few days later the salinity preference of the young salmon. Pituitary cells which produce ACTH also increase in number during the process of smoltification.

As mentioned in Chapter 5 prolactin plays an important part in the control of water and sodium movement in fresh water teleosts and appears to be the major pituitary factor necessary for fresh-water osmoregulation in the teleost fish. It is, however, difficult to establish how this ability of the hormone to conserve sodium and to reduce water flux in a number of tissues is related to the migratory process. Nevertheless there is considerable evidence which indicates that prolactin synthesis or release is controlled by environmental salinity and therefore as salmon (or elvers) move into fresh water one might expect prolactin plasma increase and/or increase in mammotrophs (prolactin-secreting cells). In fact mammotroph activity has been shown to change before or during migration into fresh water, seemingly in anticipation of the osmoregulatory challenge both in elvers and salmon. Experimentally there is a rapid significant drop in pituitary prolactin content of the coho salmon when transferred to sea water from fresh water whereas plasma prolactin levels exceed their sea-water levels after some forty hours. While it would appear that prolactin plays an active part in anadromous migration its role in catadromous migration is more problematic. The prolactin cells of the eel appear much reduced in activity when the adult eel moves from the river to the sea but plasma prolactin levels of upstream Pacific salmon can be lower than the prolactin plasma levels of fish caught out at sea.

Prolactin is involved in the migration of other species of fish such as the marine three-spined stickleback, *Gasterosteus aculeatus* (L. trachurus) and the striped mullet, *Mugil cephalus*. The stickleback lives in the sea during the autumn and winter and migrates to fresh water to breed during the spring or early summer returning to the sea in autumn after breeding. T.J. Lam has shown that during the autumn and winter prolactin synthesis appears to be inhibited, possibly by the decreasing or short daylength. As the spring approaches prolactin synthesis is triggered, possibly by increasing daylength and prolactin is stored in the pituitary in preparation for migration into fresh water. When the fish enters fresh water prolactin is released, possibly a response to lowered blood osmolality, enabling the fish to osmoregulate in its new environment. There is no evidence to imply that prolactin causes the stickleback to migrate to fresh water. The striped mullet moves from fresh water to sea water to spawn and during this annual migration changes in plasma concentration of prolactin have been observed again suggesting an osmoregulatory role for prolactin linked to migration.

There is some evidence that increased biosynthesis and release of MSH takes place at parr-smolt transformation. Behavioural changes have been linked to MSH production in higher vertebrates and it is tempting to suggest, as Fontaine has done, that the increased MSH production in the smolt plays a role in the process of attention and memorisation that the acquisition of physiological and biochemical conditions permitting homing must imply. MSH has also been shown in higher vertebrates to have a natriuretic effect and an effect on heart force and rate. Both of these effects could be useful in the process of fish migration.

The role of gonadotropin as a causal or supportive agent in fish migration has been examined, but there is no evidence to indicate any such relationships.

When the young salmon smoltifies or when the yellow eel transforms into a silver eel yet another morphological modification of an endocrine gland takes place. This is the increase in activity, judged by histological criteria, of the corpuscles of Stannius. Sexually mature Atlantic salmon in fresh water show a degranulation of the typical corpuscle cell and the appearance of a new type of cell the function of which is unknown. Long-term exposure of silver and yellow eels to either sea water or distilled water results in changes in the cells of the corpuscles of Stannius from the fresh water condition. The corpuscle of Stannius of the stickleback also modifies its cellular morphology in response to salinity. This fish has two types of cell one of which appears to be active in fresh water and the other in sea water. The hypocalcaemic hormone of the corpuscle of Stannius which lowers plasma calcium ions by changing calcium fluxes in the gill responds directly to the presence of calcium ions and therefore it is not surprising that morphological changes in the corpuscle of Stannius are associated with salinity changes. Again as in the case of prolactin the response is an osmoregulatory one and appears not causally related to migration behaviour. It has though been suggested that as neuromuscular excitability is related to the Na^+K^+/Ca^{2+} ratio then passage from fresh water to sea water may result from increased motor activity influenced by the corpuscles of Stannius.

Salmon Ranching

Salmon ranching has been defined as an aquacultural system in which juvenile fish are released to grow, unprotected, on natural foods in marine waters from which they are harvested at marketable size. The practice of releasing juvenile fish into salmon rivers is over 100 years old. However, the early attempts in hatcheries to produce ova and fry to restock rivers were generally not successful and the economic feasibility of this method of increasing the return of adult salmon to rivers was questioned. For a number of years emphasis was placed on the enhancement of natural reproduction through improved fish passages, predator control and the development of spawning channels. In the 1950s and 1960s, however, improved survival of hatchery fish was obtained through greater knowledge of disease control and feeding. With this increased number of young salmon being released into rivers and with the hope of more returns there has come about a realisation that knowledge of and control of endocrine activity of these fish might contribute to this increased return of salmon from the sea.

Mention is made in Chapter 9 (p. 224) of how coho salmon which return to rivers only once in two years might be induced by endocrine manipulation to make annual returns. Most of the applied hormonal research in salmon ranching has though been concerned with accelerating fry growth and with improving egg production and controlling ovulation.

The means by which growth may be enhanced in coho salmon in order that the optimum time for release during smoltification so that fish may commence their anadromous migration has already been discussed. Body size is critical to successful release and hormone feeding may help in achieving this. The treatment with anabolic hormones to accelerate growth generally requires two to three months. However, as the pink and chum salmon only have a fresh water feeding phase of four to six weeks and chinook salmon migrate to the sea as fry then probably only the coho salmon is a suitable ranched fish for anabolic hormone feeding. All species of Pacific and Atlantic salmon respond to anabolic androgens but the response is affected by dosage, as previously seen, by duration of application, water temperature and photoperiod and even by food ration and quality. This technique for enhancing growth has not yet become a commercial practice. Triiodothyronine, as mentioned previously, may also offer a prospect, as a growth promotor for anadromous salmonids but more importantly could be used to enhance salt water tolerance. It has been suggested that lipid reserves of salmonids at the time of their entry into sea water may influence their ocean survival and hence return. Steroid and thyroid hormones are known to alter body lipid content and composition so again there may be a considerable advantage in treating the hatchery-reared salmonid fish destined to be released with feed containing these hormones.

Obviously no hormonal treatment can be applied to hatchery-reared salmon during their year or more at sea and it is this period that would enable all traces of fed hormones and their metabolites to be eliminated prior to their return to the river estuary where they may be caught for human consumption.

With the advent of the aquaculture (sea-cage rearing) of salmon and with the increase of hatchery-produced smolts for release to sea has arisen the phenomenon of 'stunted' fish. As higher temperatures encourage better food-conversion and growth it has become common practice to rear coho salmon at a higher than ambient temperature thus reducing the period of fresh water residence to about six months. However, after transfer to sea water up to 40 percent of these fish grow very slowly if at all. These small fish have prominent parr marks in contrast with the normal silvery colour of smolts. This 'stunting' appears to have its causation in endocrine changes. These seawater-adapted parr have fewer and less active prolactin cells than normal seawater animals, more somatotrophs and regressed thyroid and endocrine pancreas glands.

If, however, these stunted fish are returned to fresh water for four months they acquire a silvery appearance, the pituitary becomes normal and many survive as smolt in sea water during the next spring as so-called 'parr-revertants'. Another change in the life history of coho salmon may be brought about by preventing smolts entering sea water in which case they undergo desmoltification and regress to parr-like pigmentation but retain many of the morphological characteristics associated with smolt.

It is not known which endocrine deficiency, if any, is the primary cause of 'stunting'. In many respects the stunt is hypo-endocrine, however, the growth hormone cells, as mentioned previously and the corpuscles of Stannius cells show signs of appreciable activity. The neurohypophysial area close to the somatotrophs is degenerated in most stunts. Plasma insulin is lower in sea water stunts than in sea water smolts and plasma concentrations of thyroxine are lower in 'parr-revertants' than in sea water smolt. However, there is no difference in plasma concentrations of triiodothyronine between sea water parr-revertants and sea water smolts. Stunts also show changes in the morphology and the biochemistry of the gill, skin, scales, muscle, liver, kidney and intestine.

Pheromones

When anadromous salmonid fishes return to fresh water to spawn after staying in the sea, they go home to their native river. As previously mentioned when discussing pheromones a sense of smell has been shown to be essential for correct homing in salmon and this must imply the presence of specific substances in each river. The pheromones hypothesis postulates that salmon smolts migrating to sea release population specific substances which form odour trails that guide the mature salmon back to their native river. If this idea can be substantiated then isolation and manipulation of pheromones could play an important part in future salmon ranching. The olfactory sensitivity of Atlantic salmon to substances emanating from their own bodies has been investigated and the intestine has been shown to contain a potent olfactory-stimulating substance. However, pheromones may not solely be olfactory guides for homing but recognition of olfactory cues inprinted during early development may play an important role as might attraction by non-specific olfactory cues. Imprinting with artificial odours such as morpholine or phenethyl alcohol results in return rates being higher than for non-imprinted fish. However, the attraction of non-imprinted salmon by these substances has also been demonstrated. It is therefore not possible at present to assess if pheromones or non-pheromone attractants play the major part in the return migration of salmon from the ocean.

9 HORMONES AND AQUACULTURE

The husbandry of aquatic organisms is an ancient practice and the culture of carp by the early Chinese dynasties and in the medieval stew-ponds of Europe is well known. However, it is only during the past quarter of a century that the art of fish culture has had modern science and technology applied to it. In the past throughout the world the culture of both fresh water and marine fish and shellfish has depended on the natural reproduction, growth, and feeding of animals in simple earth ponds and enclosures. Today though fish are farmed, as is the case with other forms of livestock, by the feeding of supplementary foodstuffs and by controlled breeding procedures.

As explained in the introduction fish endocrinology developed as a part of general and comparative endocrinology during the 1950s and during the past two decades has developed largely as an academic branch of science with little if any applied interest. Fish endocrinologists have concerned themselves with physiological and evolutionary problems and not with food production. Only during the past few years has fish endocrinology become in any sense an applied science. Now aquaculture and salmon ranching are considered a proper domain of investigation by fish endocrinologists.

Induced Spawning

There is an exception to the somewhat recent association of hormones and aquaculture, this is the practice of hormonally inducing spawning in fish. This originated in 1934 when in Brazil fish pituitary glands were injected to induce ovulation. In fact it was a famous endocrinologist, B.A. Houssay of Argentina, who in 1930 injected some small viviparous fish with pituitary glands, recently removed from another species of fish, and brought about premature birth of the young. This new finding came to the attention of R. von Ihering who was director of fish culture at Ceara in Brazil. For many years the major problem in Brazilian fish culture had been to get fish to spawn in captivity; even if they were caught nearly ripe they rarely completed maturity or ovulated. By 1934 von Ihering had developed a successful technique for inducing ovulation using fish pituitaries. This process is sometimes now known as hypophysation.

During this period the Russians had been attempting to induce captive sturgeon to ripen and spawn by means of mammalian hormones but it was not until 1937 that N.L. Gerbil'skii was able to obtain ripe eggs and sperm from a significant number of sturgeon, *Acipenser stellatus*, that had been intraperitoneally injected with one or two fresh pituitaries from fish of the same species. This was a fortunate discovery, because at this time hydroelectric stations and dams were being built on the rivers which sturgeon used for upstream spawning thus preventing the sturgeon reaching their sites of ovulation. With the technique of hypophysation fish could be spawned near the mouth of the river. Today the Russians obtain all sturgeon eggs for culturing from pituitary treated fish.

It was in the early 1950s that induced spawning of carp in China and in India began to be practiced widely. In China the black carp, *Mylopharyngodon piceus*, and the big head, *Aristichthys nobilis*, were first induced to spawn by pituitary injection, then silver carp, *Hypophthalmichthys molitrix* and finally grass carp, *Ctenopharyngodon idellus*. In India it has been the major carps, the catla, *Catla catla*, the rohu, *Labeo rohita*, and the mrigal, *Cirrhinus mrigala*, that have been spawned intensively with the aid of pituitary hormones.

It must be remembered that pituitary extracts are not used to induce gonadal development but only to initiate ovulation. Once resorption of eggs has begun then the process of pituitary gland injection will not reverse the situation. Most of the Chinese carps respond to pituitary preparations from many different kinds of animals but the Indian carp respond with more species specificity to pituitaries taken from fully mature ripe fish. The generally accepted dosage for big head, black carp and silver carp are 2 to 3 mg of dried cyprinid pituitary or three fresh glands. Grass carp require a slighly higher dose. Normally a small priming dose is injected (one-eighth of total) and then some 6 to 24 hours later the remainder of the pituitary material is injected. After this time natural spawning or stripping for artificial insemination may take place. Major carps generally receive a priming dose of 2-3 mg of pituitary/kg body weight then after six hours a second dose of 6-8 mg/kg body weight. Males receive only one dose. For both Chinese and Indian carp breeding fish generally of several kilograms in weight have to be selected for maturity before pituitary injection. Maturity of males is more easily determined, fully mature animals ooze milt when the abdomen is gently pressed, but females are more difficult to sex although soft rounded bulging abdomens and swollen reddish vents are external indicators of maturity.

The technique described for Chinese and Indian carp is similarly applied to other species of fish although the dosage of pituitary injected and details of the technique vary. For example induced spawning of the Channel catfish is widely practised with carp pituitary being used. The dose needed to induce spawning is about 13 mg/kg body weight. Spawning of mullet has been induced by the injection of ripe females with several types of preparations including salmon pituitary, carp pituitary and various mammalian pituitary preparations. Mature mullet are more difficult to determine than carp and the stages of the development of oocytes cannot be determined by any convenient method of external examination. Therefore, a cannula is inserted into the oviduct and a few oocytes withdrawn for determination of maturity stages prior to pituitary injection. The common carp, *Cyprinus carpio,* is induced to breed by the use of pituitary gland injections throughout the world particularly in temperate regions when brood fish may be brought up to the required temperature for gonad maturation (20°C) and subsequent pituitary injection and spawning carried out at any time of the year. This allows the fish farmer to schedule his work rigidly and to provide fry throughout the year. The dose of pituitary required for this species is 2-3 mg/kg body weight of an acetone-dried preparation. Although, as has been implied, most species of fish which have been given pituitary extracts respond to material from unrelated species the common carp has thus far been found to respond only to pituitary extracts of its own species.

As is seen from the above the effects of exogenous pituitary preparations on ovulation in a number of teleosts have been investigated and farming practices established over a period of many years. However, the use of pituitary preparations in salmonids in order to obtain fertilised ova at an earlier date, to synchronise hatchery production or to reduce pre-spawning mortality has not yet been established even though as early as 1939 Hasler successfully induced ovulation in trout using carp pituitary. The reason for this is probably that as salmonids are annual, or one time only, spawners induced spawning is less commercially desirable or necessary. Nevertheless, crude salmon pituitary extract has been shown to induce the final maturation and ovulation of coho salmon over the entire normal spawning period. More purified preparations of salmon pituitary have been shown to induce ovulation in the Ayu (*Plecoglossus altivelis*). Also in order to obtain simultaneous ovulation of Danube salmon (*Hucho hucho*), all females within a hatching stock have been injected with carp pituitary giving positive results.

A potential that exists in aquaculture is the growing of eels from egg to maturation in a culture situation. For this to occur mature and spawning brood fish must be produced. Injection of acetone-dried pituitary glands have been given to Japanese eels and mature eggs have been produced. Fertilisation has been achieved and larvae develop normally for a short while before dying. Perhaps in the future these larvae will grow to a harvestable size.

Although mainly pituitary hormones have been used in aquaculture to induce spawning other hormones and drugs have been investigated and used. Human chorionic gonadotropin (HCG) is a glycoprotein produced by the placenta and appears in the urine during early pregnancy in large quantities. Although HCG is found normally only in pregnant women it produces a great variety of gonadal action in many other vertebrates. In a number of species of fish it may cause release of spermatozoa and ova from the mature gonads possibly acting synergistically with circulating endogenous gonadotropins of pituitary origin. This possibility tends to be verified by the fact that HCG when injected with fish pituitary extracts produces a better response in fish than when the preparations are given singly. HCG being relatively cheap can be applied in those situations in aquaculture where a fish is refractory to all but its own pituitary and when the pituitary costs are high or availability of pituitary extract limited.

11-Desoxycorticosterone-acetate (DOCA) has been used to induce maturation of oocytes in females of Clariid species from many parts of the world. Broodfish are selected by the injection of the hormone and the females can be stripped by hand. The catfish, *Heteropneustes fossilis*, also ovulates in response to DOCA. Ovulation may also be induced in salmonids by a single injection of 17α-hydroxy-20β-dihydroprogesterone which is a natural steroid occurring at high concentrations in female salmon plasma at the time of spawning and is probably a natural mediator of oocyte

maturation. *In vivo* this steroid can, when injected into females
having oocytes with the germinal vesicle in the subperipheral
position induce the full sequence of oocyte maturation and ovulation. Due to the cost of production there is little likelihood of this
steroid being used commercially for egg production. The anti-
oestrogen tamoxifen (1-[p-(β-dimethylaminoethoxy) phenyl]-1,
2-transdiphenyl but-l-ene) has been used in conjunction with a
pituitary extract primer to induce early ovulation in coho salmon
(Figure 9.1). The anti-androgen is thought to exert its influence on
the hypothalamus and gonadotropin release. This drug must be
regarded as a research tool rather than a commercial product for
inducing ovulation. Finally mention should be made of how ovulation may be induced by LH-RH and LH-RH analogues. Ovulation has been induced by synthetic luteinising hormone and
release hormone (LH-RH) in a number of teleost fish (Figure 9.2)
and also in the coho salmon two nonapeptide analogues have been
shown to accelerate the ovulation process (Figure 9.3). Unfortunately although LH-RH and its analogues are relatively cheap to
produce there is rapid clearance of these polypeptides and there
will be need to devise long-acting forms before release factors have
any possible role in aquaculture.

Although fish pituitary extracts, particularly carp, are very
widely used throughout the world to induce ovulation there is no
reason to suppose that if ovulatory substances could be produced
sufficiently cheaply they would not replace pituitary material.

Sexual Maturity and Sterility

Although the vast majority of concern with hormones and reproduction has been with the induction of egg and sperm production
both the production of precocious sexual maturation and the inhibition of gonadal development are relevant to aquaculture.

The pink salmon, *Oncorhynchus gorbuscha*, of Western
Canada is peculiar in that it has a rigid two-year life cycle so that in
some rivers no salmon spawn in alternate years. If the fish could be
induced to spawn one year earlier then the rivers which are normally devoid of fish in the second year could become stocked. It
has been possible to accelerate sexual maturation in male pink
salmon by intraperitoneal injection of partially purified salmon
gonadotropin so that milt is produced one year earlier than

Figure 9.1: Induced Ovulation of Coho Salmon (*Oncorhynchus kisutch*). The number of fish which ovulated in the two groups administered a priming injection of 0.1 mg/kg SG-G100 followed by a second injection of 1.0 or 10.0 mg/kg tamoxifen and the peanut oil control are expressed as a cumulative percentage of their respective groups. Arrows indicate the days on which the injections were administered. The normal peak spawning period for Big Qualicum coho is 20-25 November.

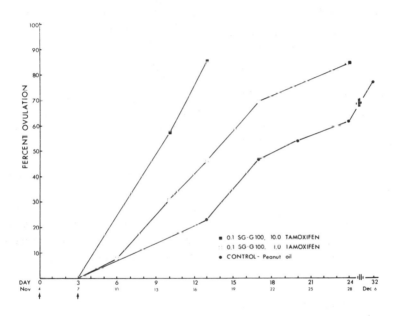

Source: Donaldson, E.M., Hunter, G.A. and Dye, H.M. (1981/82) Induced ovulation in coho salmon (*Oncorhynchus kisutch*). III. Preliminary study on the use of the antiestrogen tamoxifen. *Aquaculture, 26,* 143-54.

normal but it has not yet been possible to obtain female pink salmon which approach sexual maturity until the January of the year in which they would normally spawn. Although it may be possible to improve the ranching of this salmon by accelerating maturity the need to produce precociously mature fish generally in aquaculture seems very remote.

A more widely required economic need in fish farming might be to prevent gonadal maturation. The idea of improved conversion

Figure 9.2: Dose-Response Relationships of LH-RH on Induction of Ovulation in Four Teleosts: Ayu, *Plecoglossus altivelis* (data from Hirose and Ishida 1974b; Goldfish, *Carassius auratus*: Plaice, *Limanda yokohamae*, and Goby *Acanthogobius flavimanus*.

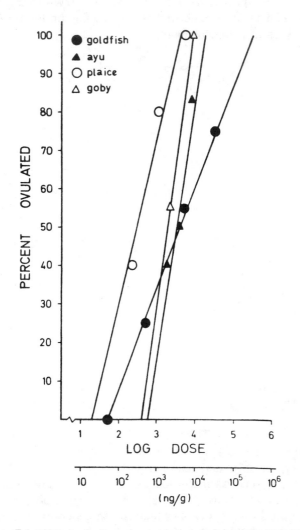

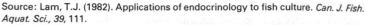

Source: Lam, T.J. (1982). Applications of endocrinology to fish culture. *Can. J. Fish. Aquat. Sci., 39*, 111.

Figure 9.3: Induced Ovulation of Coho Salmon (*Oncorhynchus kisutch*). The numbers of fish which ovulated in the saline control and the groups administered a 0.1 mg/kg SG-G100 primer followed by three injections of 1.6 mg/kg LH-RH or 0.2 mg/kg D-Ala^6 analogue are expressed as cumulative percentages of their respective groups. Arrows indicate the days on which the injections were administered. The normal peak spawning period for Big Qualicum coho is 20-25 November.

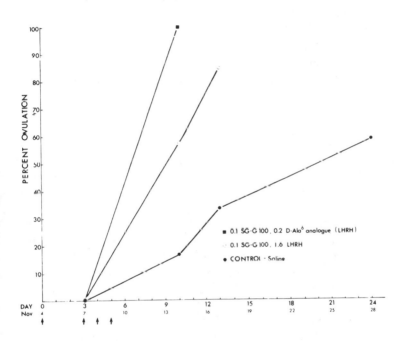

Source: Donaldson, E.M., Hunter, G.A. and Dye, H.M. (1981/2) Induced ovulation in coho salmon (*Oncorhynchus kisutch*). II. Preliminary study of the use of LH-RH and two high potency LH-RH analogues. *Aquaculture, 26*, 129-41.

of food into flesh with no wastage by conversion of food into gonad material is one which has appealed to many farmers. Also in salmonid species cessation of somatic growth is accompanied by the flesh becoming watery and an increased susceptibility of animals to fungal disease. It is for all these reasons, particularly in salmonids that experiments have been made in order to establish the possibility and commercial viability of producing asexual fish.

Sterilisation by surgical gonadectomy has been successfully carried out on salmonids with low mortality. Commercially though the method is not suitable because of the time required for the operation and the fact that the operation can only be performed on fish above a certain size. Also in some countries the operation may be performed only by veterinary surgeons. Sex steroid hormones can also be used to inhibit gonadal development and spermatogenesis. However, results obtained so far are erratic. Steroids given by intraperitoneal injection in the diet, or by immersion of juveniles before or at the time of sex differentiation sometimes induces sterilisation but not inevitably. Sometimes spermatogenesis is even stimulated.

An investigation of the inhibitory effect of some steroids on spermatogenesis in adult rainbow trout, *Salmo gairdneri,* was made by Billard and his colleagues. Various sex steroids were fed at doses of 0.05 and 0.5 mg/kg food. The high dose of oestradiol-17β and the low dose of methyltestosterone totally inhibited testicular growth. However, only partial inhibition occurred using testosterone. Also these inhibitions only occured when the hormones were administered during the summer. No change in plasma gonadotropin occurred after male sex hormone treatment indicating that the steroids act directly at the level of the gonad. The use of exogenous steroids to inhibit gametogenesis in salmonids does not appear at the moment to be a technique for producing sterile fish which is a reliable one although in some species high steroid doses result in gonad inhibition if given to the young. Also the fact that hormones have to be fed to fish that will be used for human consumption raises the problem of undesirable chemical residues being present in the fish when they are eaten.

Another technique that has been investigated for the inhibition of gonad maturation has been the treatment of fish with non-hormonal non-steroid chemicals which inhibit pituitary gonadotropin activity and are thus anti-androgenic. Two chemical compounds that have been investigated widely are methallibure (1α-methylallyl-thiocarbamoyl-2-methylthiocarbamoyl-hydrazine, ICI, UK) and cyproterone acetate (2α-methylene-6-chloro-pregnadiene-17α- ol-3, 20-dione α-acetate). Although both these drugs reduce gonadotropin production and lower androgen secretion they do not prevent gonad maturation. Possibly to be effective as chemosterilants these chemicals might have to be administered in the diet of young fry but again as with the use of steroids as sterilants there would bound to be public concern if these drugs were used commercially in aquaculture to improve the growth and fattening of farmed fish.

Although there is no endocrine connection another method of producing sterility in fish which may show promise in aquaculture should be mentioned. It is the induction of triploidy by prevention of the dissociation of the second polar body in the egg. This is generally carried out by temperature shock and these triploid-induced fish show impaired gonad development. However this impairment of growth varies both between the sexes and from species to species.

Single Sex Fish Culture (Monosex Culture)

It has already been mentioned that sterilised fish converting the bulk of their ingested energy into flesh and not into gonad development might have advantages in aquaculture. This procedure is not easy to adopt commercially but another approach may be to produce either all males or all females depending upon which sex has the better conversion efficiency and growth rate. Another disadvantage in the culture of some fish such as tilapia is that they are very fecund and are able to reproduce at a relatively small size causing overpopulation of ponds with fish that are less than a harvestable size. Single sex culture would prevent this.

There are three ways in which unwanted spawning can be controlled. First, the fish might be sexed before maturity and the males and females reared separately or the faster growing sex reared solely. Secondly, particularly as in the case of tilapia different species might be crossed and for some unknown reason progeny of nearly all males can often be produced. Thirdly fry can be fed on a minute amount of sex hormones and all male or all female broods produced. Sexing fish by eye is difficult for young fish show no sexual dimorphism while hybridisation rarely results in 100 per cent males in tilapia. In both these methods there is no certainty of monosex culture production. Only hormone treatment of fry has any reliability for the production of single sex fish stocks and then only if the treatment is made with the correct dose at the correct time and for the correct length of time.

All developing vertebrate gonads pass through a stage when

they contain tissue for differentiation into both testes and ovary. In most vertebrates there is a differentiation of this tissue into two rudiments, the medulla, which normally gives rise to testes and an outer cortex region which gives rise to the ovary. However, in teleost fish there is no such distinct organisation, the potential male and female tissue is intermingled and this indifferent gonadal tissue can readily be triggered to form either definitive ovary or testes by hormonal treatment. Much research has taken place into the problem of sex differentiation and to the question of what are the factors which induce undifferentiated tissue to become male or female germ cell producing organs. However, for our purposes it is not necessary to be so concerned but merely to realise that the gonadal anlage in most teleosts is very labile and can be directed into producing either a functional male or female gonad by exogenous hormone treatment.

Sex reversal in both directions was first acheived by Yamamoto in the medaka fish, *Oryzias latipes*, and later in the goldfish, *Carassius auratus*. Complete sex reversals were obtained by the administration of gonadal hormones to the juveniles of genetically analysed breeds. Yamamoto also demonstrated that in addition to the early gonads having the ability to differentiate in a direction opposite to their own genetic constitution, the genetic complement of the germ cells is not altered by the procedures employed in producing the reversal of sex.

Since this time sex reversal has been accomplished in many species of fish. Because of the fact that small tilapia breed indiscriminately, that the male of this species grows faster than the female and that the species is of great commercial interest means that sex reversal is important in this species. Methyltestosterone in doses of 15-60 mg/kg food have been used to produce an all-male population. The drug is given during the first 30-50 days of life during the period when the gonadal differentiation of tilapia takes place. Another synthetic androgen, ethynyltestosterone has also been used to induce sex reversal in tilapia. Generally the use of oestrogenic steroids to alter the sex of fishes has been less successful than the efforts with androgens and the effects of oestrogenic hormones such as oestrone, oestriol, oestradiol and diethylstilboestrol on primary and secondary sex characteristics differ widely in various species. In treatment of tilapia with oestrogens a 100 per cent sex reversal has not been obtained. However, recently it has been reported that sex-reversal females of *Tilapia aurea* can be produced if fry shorter than 13 mm are fed for six weeks with a diet containing 17α- ethynyloestradiol and methallibure each at a concentration of 100 mg/kg food.

Although the production of sex-reversed females is not yet practised commercially all male populations are produced. For example in Israel *Tilapia aurea* are spawned naturally, the spawning fish removed from the ponds and the newly hatched fry collected for hormone treatment. The fry are then placed in large tanks fed with a diet containing methyltestosterone for five weeks and the fish all male are then sold or grown on. By this method in one year between 3000 and 5000 male fry are produced from one female.

Although the interest in sex reversal in salmonid culture was not generated until after that of tilapia the potential of rearing single sex stocks for more efficient farming is enormous. Unlike the situation with tilapia it is the female of the species which is more highly valued. Male salmonids as previously mentioned on reaching maturity develop a number of adverse characteristics such as deterioration of flesh quality, pigmentation of skin and in the case of salmon form grilse more readily than females. The problems associated with maturity would become unimportant in trout or would be reduced in salmon culture if all female stocks of fish could be produced.

The first attempts to feminise salmonids by exogenous steroid hormone treatment were largely unsuccessful. However, the oral administration of 17β-oestradiol at concentrations of 20 mg/kg food to juvenile rainbow trout and Atlantic salmon for periods of up to 60 days induces sex reversal amongst the males and results in all-female stocks whose gonads are indistinguishable histologically from normal females.

Using techniques similar to that used for Atlantic salmon, Pacific salmon, *Oncorhynchus* sp. have been used also for the production of all-female stocks. However, the treatment needs to be commenced at the eyed egg stage and to be continued through the alevin and feeding stages. Immersion of the fish in the drug as well as feeding appears to be necessary to bring about sex reversal here. After immersion of eyed eggs in oestradiol (400µg/l) it has been shown that very low doses of oestradiol (2-5 mg/kg food) need to be fed to bring about 100 per cent feminisation. Obviously from the points of both drug expense and drug consumption risk this technique has advantage.

Although direct feminisation by oestradiol is the easiest way to obtain all-female stocks an indirect technique has been developed which is now being used by trout farmers. Genetically female fish are converted into functional males by feeding methyltestosterone (3 mg/kg food) to first-feeding fry for about two months. The sex-reversal males have no Wolffian ducts but produce milt which is used to ferilise normal eggs. As no Y chromosomes are present in the sperm (the normal male trout is heterogamic) then females only will be produced after artificial fertilisation. This method still produces females which convert much of their energy intake into ovarian tissue. Sterile fish do not. In order to produce sterile fish these all-female stock produced from the sperm of hormonally masculinised females could have their eggs subjected to a heat shock so that all-female triploid fish are produced. These female triploid fish show virtually no gonad development. This technique of producing sterile triploid females by combining the techniques of producing triploids with hormonal masculinisation could be a commercial advantage for the future.

Stress

During the past twenty years with the advent of intensive farming, particularly in North America and Europe, the fact that fish were reared in densities far exceeding those found in nature, were transported in confined environments, were handled for stripping and spawning purposes, were forced through grading machines and subject to other husbandry pressures inevitably led fish farmers and biologists to think about stress. Both for the layman and the scientist the concept of biological stress has been a difficult one to define; even Hans Selye, a pioneer and outstanding worker in the field originally defined stress in terms of the applied stimulus but later re-defined it as a biological response and the stimulus as the stressor.

In spite of the arguments regarding the definition and terminology of the stress phenomenon (Is stress an essential part of normal metabolism?) the aquaculturist has taken an empirical and pragmatic view of stress defining the phenomenon as those unusual activities that take place when animals are crowded and directed to move against their will, handled or subjected to pollution or chemical change in the water. Thus stress to the majority of fish farmers means the response measured in terms of increased activity, increased ventilation, increased mortality and increased susceptibility to disease.

Central to the definition of stress by the scientist is the concept of Selye that a wide variety of stress stimulations bring about a common response. This response is furthermore divided on a temporal basis into the stages of alarm, resistance and exhaustion. However, these stages may vary enormously in their strength and duration in response to different stimuli. Fish have been shown to respond to stress in a manner similar to that shown by higher vertebrates and appear to show similar neural and neuroendocrine primary responses. It is with these neuroendocrine and subsequent endocrine changes that take place during the stress response that the fish endocrinologist is particularly concerned. As stress may be considered as an environmental factor which reduces the ability of a fish to maintain homeostasis and to carry out normal growth and reproduction it is to be expected that many endocrine glands will be affected.

A change in catecholamines, as occurring in mammals, was looked for and found following stress stimulations. A 'flight and fight' response has thus been established in fish associated with very high levels of adrenaline (Chapter 4). Also many of the metabolic effects brought about by catecholamines are seen in the stressed fish. Elevation of blood glucose and blood lactic acid and breakdown of muscle glycogen occur. It is, however, difficult to distinguish the primary catecholamine stress response and its metabolic effects from another hormonal response, namely that of corticosteroid production following a stress stimulus. Both interrenal cells and chromaffin cells are activated by stress stimuli and the products of both these cells cause elevation of plasma blood glucose. Cortisol levels in the blood rise rapidly after handling and netting with these high values often not returning to normal for many days. Although perhaps the cortisol parameter of the brain-pituitary-interrenal axis is the easiest to measure, and has been most widely cited in stress experiments, other parameters such as ACTH, interrenal ascorbic acid levels and cytological measurements can all be used to show that this axis is profoundly affected by stress.

Although the handling procedures used in aquaculture, particularly in the rearing of salmonids in raceways or tanks, all bring about elevation of plasma cortisol levels these levels may also be elevated by other intensive fish husbandry technology. For example changes in oxygen concentration, free ammonia concentration, pH and salinity changes have all been shown to elevate plasma cortisol levels. Again pesticides, heavy metals, contaminants in artificial foods may all act as stress stimuli. Although it is of interest to note here that no significant effects of cadmium on the plasma cortisol levels of the coho salmon, *Oncorhynchus kisutch*, were observed even though the metal was present at levels that were ultimately lethal. Finally, diseases which are endemic to certain fish cultures, such as myxobacteria infection, bacterial kidney disease and saprolegnia fungal infection all appear to cause elevation of plasma cortisol.

In spite of considerable laboratory and experimental work indicating the response of the chromaffin tissue and the hypothalamic-pituitary-interrenal axis to stress stimuli very little has been done to use these changes in hormonal levels either to quantify and compare the relative significance of different stresses or to predict the necessity of modifying an aquacultural procedure.

Other hormone levels which appear to vary under a stress stimulus are thyroid hormones, prolactin, angiotensin and the neurohypophysial peptides, vasotocin and isotocin. It would also be surprising if growth hormone changes did not take place in response to stress stimuli. When farmed rainbow trout are transported it has been noted that thyroxine and triiodothyronine concentrations in the blood fall by over 75 per cent. Normal values were regained by TSH injections.

Perhaps stress stimuli stimulate the TSH-inhibiting factor of the hypothalamus, but that must be conjecture. Prolactin undoubtedly plays a part in the stress response brought about by salinity changes. As it is a hormone important in hydromineral balance maintaining the homeostasis of membrane permeability to ions and water, then alterations in salinity will influence plasma prolactin levels. The role of this hormone is probably as important as the corticosteroids and catecholamines in circumstances when the stress stimulus induces any osmoregulatory imbalance.

Growth Promotion and Feeding

A primary aim of fish farming is to obtain faster tissue growth more economically. Efforts to improve the efficiency of food conversion have occupied aquacultural scientists for a number of years. The fact that anabolic promoting drugs had been used in animal husbandry to enhance growth rate and realise substantial savings in production costs prompted investigations into the use of such sex hormones and their synthetic analogues in fish. Early experiments where the hormones were injected were obviously unsuited to commercial exploitation. The hormonal growth pro-motors to be used in fish farming must be incorporated into the feed.

McBride and Fagerlund in 1973 reported on the use of methyltestosterone for promoting weight increase in juvenile Pacific salmon while Simpson and his colleagues in 1974 were the first to show that rainbow trout and Atlantic salmon parr when fed with a diet supplemented with either ethyloestranol or methyl-testosterone exhibited a significant increase in growth and an improvement of food conversion efficiency. Since that time many hormones have been investigated as potential anabolic agents. Diethylstilboestrol which has been widely used in animal husbandry and although not a steroid has oestrogenic properties, is without effect in fish. Also trenbolone acetate (17β-acetoxy-3-oxoestra-4, 9, 11-triene) a derivation of testosterone is without effect in carp. However, a number of anabolic steroids both androgenic and oestrogenic do increase growth and food conversion efficiency when administered in food. Foremost among these as previously mentioned is 17α-methyltestosterone. In carp 2.5-5.0 ppm is the optimum dose for growth and at concentrations above 5.0 ppm there is no induction of significant growth, the hormone tending to be catabolic at these higher doses. Fish receiving up to 5.0 ppm of the hormone are several hundred per cent heavier than their con-trols after three months of treatment. Nearly all species of Pacific salmon have been shown to increase growth when fed methyl-testosterone (Figure 9.4) and in all species so far tested methyl-testosterone appears to be the most potent of the anabolic steroids in fish. Nevertheless, a number of other steroids such as dimethazine (2α-17α- dimethyl-17β-hydroxy-5α-androstan-3,3'-azine) stano-zolol (17β-hydroxy-17α-methyl-5-androstano-(3,2-C)-pyrazole), ethyloestrenol (17β-hydroxy-17α-ethyloestra-4 en-3-one) and norethandrolone (17α-ethyl-17β-hydroxy-19-norandrost-4-enone) significantly increase weight gain in fish (carp and salmonids) when incorporated in the diet (Figure 9.5).

Figure 9.4: Mean Weights of Coho Salmon Receiving 17α-methyltestosterone-supplemented Diets While Maintained in Freshwater of 11.5° and 16.5°C.

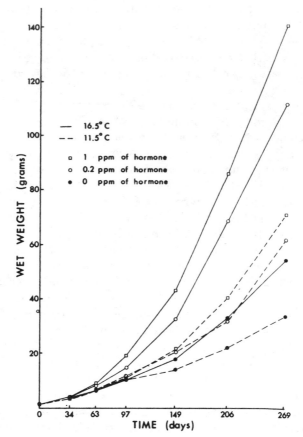

Source: Fagerlund, U.H.M. and McBride, J.R. (1977) The effect of 17α-methyltestosterone on growth, gonadal development, external features and proximate composition of muscle of steelhead trout, coho and pink salmon. *Fish. Mar. Serv. Tech. Rep.* no. *716.*

All the compounds mentioned above, including methyl-testosterone are synthetic compounds, however, naturally occurring androgens and oestrogens are anabolic. In fish testosterone and 11-ketotestosterone are naturally occurring androgens whereas adrenosterone (4-androsten-3,11,17-trione) is a metabolic product of natural androgens in fish. These three compounds

Figure 9.5: The Effect of Feeding Ethyloestrenol on Weight of the Carp, *Cyprinus carpio*. Arrow indicates discontinuation of hormone feed.

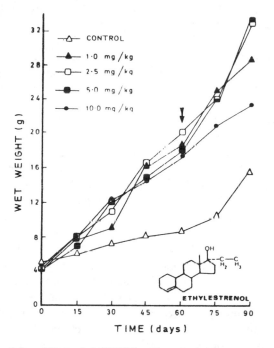

Source: Lone, K.P. and Matty, A.J. (1983) The effect of ethylestrenol on the growth, food conversion and tissue chemistry of the carp, *Cyprinus carpio*. *Aquaculture, 32,* 39-55.

have been fed to the carp, *Cyprinus carpio,* and have been shown to increase growth and food conversion efficiency. Oestrogens unlike androgens when administered in food to fish do not enhance growth but often result in negative growth. Oestrogens, therefore, appear unsuited as growth promotors in fish food.

Theoretically growth hormone could be used as a growth enhancing agent in fish culture. However, there are two major factors that mitigate against its use, first the difficulty of obtaining sufficient quantities and secondly as a polypeptide one would expect the hormone to be destroyed by digestive enzymes if given orally. Therefore its use in aquaculture appears limited. However, the possibility lies in the future of the biotechnological synthesis of the molecule. Also it may be possible to administer the hormone orally as there is an indication that growth may be enhanced after oral feeding. It could be possible that the molecule before absorption may be only partially cleaved, as may be the case with bovine growth hormone, fragments of which when digested retain some growth promoting activity. Although oral feeding of growth hormone seems a scenario for the future it is now perfectly feasible to enhance growth by injection or implantation of the hormone (Figure 9.6). The use of bovine growth hormone in this manner could be used for the rapid growing on of selected stock for breeding purposes.

Although insulin has a part to play in nitrogen retention by fish, like growth hormone its use in aquaculture seems remote and for much the same reasons. The only other candidates for use in aquaculture are the thyroid hormones. Although early reports on the growth-promoting ability of thyroid hormones in fish were equivocal in the past few years careful studies have established the growth enhancing and protein anabolic role of thyroxine and thiiodothyronine in fish. Careful oral application of the hormones (or analogues) in the right dose could result in a commercial future for these hormones in aquaculture. Mammalian thyroid powder, minced bovine thyroid or iodinated casein mixed into fish food have all been shown to enhance growth of Atlantic salmon, rainbow trout, guppies and swordtails. However, set against this, these treatments appear to have little or no effect on other species. In order to explain these discrepancies it has been suggested that optimum environmental or experimental conditions have not always been achieved. For example in experiments where temperature or ration are altered positive growth promotion may be achieved under one set of conditions but not under another. Oral presentation is probably not suitable for the administration of thyroxine which is poorly absorbed by the gut and which binds easily to dietary constituents reducing its likelihood of absorption. However, triiodothyronine, in doses as low as 4ppm, incorporated in the food of underyearling coho salmon results in enhancement of growth. Triiodothyroxine also when fed to rainbow trout at a dose of 5ppm, increases the feeding rate and accelerates growth. These studies point to the possibility of the use of thyroid hormones as growth promotors in aquaculture.

In all these studies on the use of hormones or hormone analogues as potential growth promotors the question that is in all investigators' minds — will residues or the hormones themselves be

Figure 9.6: Semilogarithmic Plot of Geometric Means for Wet Weights of Yearling Coho Salmon at 10°C Administered Either Bovine Growth Hormone (bGH), L-Thyroxine (T_4), 17α-methyltestosterone (MT), Combinations of These Hormones, or No Hormone (C) for 59 Days. A bar through the geometric mean denotes the 95% confidence interval. Each point is a mean of 56-60 fish.

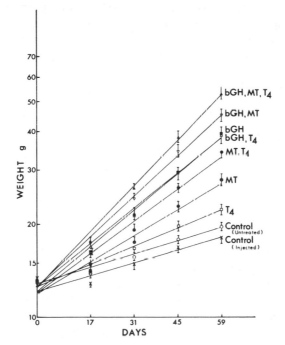

Source: Higgs, D.A. *et al.* (1977). Influence of combinations of bovine growth hormone, 17α-methyltestosterone, and L-thyroxine on growth of yearling coho salmon (*Oncorhynchus kisutch*). *Can. J. Zool.*, *55*, 1048-56.

present in the fish when they are consumed? Before there is any commercial application a suitable protocol will have to be followed that will ensure that all the residues of the drugs have been removed from the fish.

Experiments that have been carried out both on Pacific salmon and on carp using [³H]-methyltestosterone and [³H]-testosterone have shown that there is rapid elimination of these compounds. In the case of Coho salmon parr when the steroids were fed in concentrations used to promote growth residues of less than 1 ng/g

(= 1ppb) remained in the tissues ten days after the last feeding. This is much lower than the normal level of androgens found in the plasma of salmon. A similar rate of drug clearance has been shown for carp. After 12 days of [^{3}H]-testosterone feeding the radio-activity in the muscle was 10.5 ng/g and 20 days after drug with-drawal 3.8 ng/g. Again this concentration is lower than normal blood plasma values. From these and other studies it would seem that androgens could be used in fish culture for fish to be used for human consumption provided that a hormone withdrawal period was imposed (Figure 9.7). However, the law in many countries regarding permissible tissue levels of drugs is ill-defined and mini-mal levels required have tended to reflect the current limits of analytical detection.

Figure 9.7: Decline in Whole Body Levels of Orally Administered [7(n)-^{3}H] 17-MT in Tilapia and Rainbow Trout.

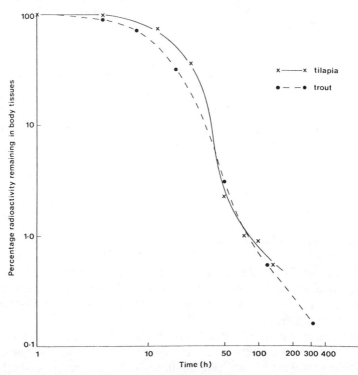

Source: Johnstone, R., Macintosh, D.J. and Wright, R.S. (1983). Elimination of orally administered 17α-methyltestosterone by *Oreochromis mossambicus* (tilapia) and *Salmo gairdneri* (rainbow trout) juveniles. *Aquaculture, 35,* 249-57.

BIBLIOGRAPHY

As explained in the introduction these suggestions for further reading are selective and relate mainly to reviews or research papers which in the author's opinion provide key points and material in the growth of the subject and contribute to the further understanding of fish endocrinology.

General

Barrington, E.J.W. (1975) *General and Comparative Endocrinology*. Oxford University Press, London.
Barrington, E.J.W. (ed.) (1979) *Hormones and Evolution*. Academic Press, New York and London.
Bentley, P.J. (1984) *Comparative Vertebrate Endocrinology* (2nd end). Cambridge University Press.
Bond, C.E. (1979) *Biology of Fishes*. W.B. Saunders, Philadelphia.
Fontaine, Y. (1975) 'Hormones in Fishes' in D. C. Malins and J.R. Sargent (eds.), *Biochemical and Biophysical Perspectives in Marine Biology*, Vol. 2. Academic Press, New York and London, p. 139.
Frieden, E. and Lipner, H. (1971) *Biochemical Endocrinology of the Vertebrates*. Prentice-Hall, Englewood Cliffs, New Jersey.
Gaillard, P.J. and Boer, H.H. (eds.) (1978) *Comparative Endocrinology*. Elsevier/North Holland, Amsterdam.
Gorbman, A. and Bern, H.A. (1962) *A Textbook of Comparative Endocrinology*. John Wiley, New York.
Greenwood, P.H., Miles, R.S. and Patterson, C. (eds.) (1973) *Interrelationships of Fishes*. Academic Press, New York.
Highnam, K.C. and Hill, L. (1969) *The Comparative Endocrinology of the Invertebrates*. Edward Arnold, London.
Hoar, W.S. and Randall, D.J. (eds.) (1969-1983) *Fish Physiology* (9 volumes). Academic Press, New York and London.
Idler, D.R. (ed.) (1972) *Steroids in Nonmammalian Vertebrates*. Academic Press, New York and London.
Lagler, K.F., Bardach, J.E., Miller, R.R. and Passino, D.R.M. (1977) *Ichthyology* (2nd edn). John Wiley, New York.
Miller, P.J. (ed.) (1979) *Fish Phenology: Anabolic Adaptiveness in Teleosts*. Symp. Zool. Soc. London No. 44, Academic Press, New York and London.
Rankin, J.C., Pitcher, T.J. and Duggan, R. (eds.) (1983) *Control Processes in Fish Physiology*. Croom Helm, London/Wiley, New York.
Turner, C.D. and Bagnara, J.T. (1971) *General Endocrinology* (5th edn). W.B. Saunders, Philadelphia.
Vincent, S. (1924) *Internal Secretions and the Ductless Glands*. Edward Arnold, London.
Nelson, J.S. (1976) *Fishes of the World*. Wiley-Interscience, New York.

Chapter 1: The Pituitary

Ball, J.N. (1969) 'Prolactin and Osmoregulation in Teleost Fishes: Review', *Gen. Comp. Endocrinol.*, Suppl. 2.

Ball, J.N. and Baker, B.I. (1969) 'The Pituitary Gland: Anatomy and Histophysiology' in W.S. Hoar and D.J. Randall (eds.), *Fish Physiology* Vol. 2, Academic Press, New York and London, p. 1.

Breton, B., Prunet, P. and Reinaud, P. (1978) 'Sexual Differences in Salmon Gonadotropin', *Ann. Biol. Anim. Bioch. Biophys.*, *18*, 759.

Chan, D.K.O. (1977) 'Comparative Physiology of the Vasomotor Effects of Neurohypophysial Peptides in the Vertebrates', *Am. Zool.*, *17*, 751.

Chang, Y. and Huang, F. (1982) 'The Mode of Action of Carp Gonadotropin on the Stimulation of Androgen Production by Carp Testis *in vitro*', *Gen. Comp. Endocrinol.*, *48*, 147.

Clarke, W.C., Farmer, S.W. and Hartwell, K.M. (1977) 'Effect of Teleost Pituitary Growth Hormone on Growth of *Tilapia mossambica* and on Growth and Seawater Adaptation of Sockeye Salmon (*Oncorhynchus nerka*)', *Gen. Comp. Endocrinol.*, *33*, 174.

Cook, A.F., Wilson S.W. and Peter, R.E. (1983) 'Development and Validation of a Carp Growth Hormone Radioimmunoassay', *Gen. Comp. Endocrinol.*, *50*, 335.

Crim, J.W., Dickoff, W.W. and Gorbman, A. (1978) 'Comparative Endocrinology of Piscine Hypothalamic Hypophysiotropic Peptides: Distribution and Activity', *Am. Zool.*, *18*, 411.

de Beer, G.R. (1926) *The Comparative Anatomy, Histology and Development of the Pituitary Body.* Oliver and Boyd, Edinburgh.

Dodd, J.M., Dodd., M.H.I., Sumpter, J.P. and Jenkins, N. (1982) 'Gonadotropic Activity in the Buccal Lobe of the Pituitary of the Rabbit Fish, *Hydrolagus Colliei*', *Gen. Comp. Endocrinol.*, *48*, 174.

Farmer, S.W., Hayashida, T., Papkoff, H. and Polenov, A.L. (1981) 'Characteristics of Growth Hormone Isolated from Sturgeon (*Acipenser guldenstadt*) pituitaries', *Endocrinology*, *108*, 377.

Fernholm, B. (1972) 'The Ultrastructure of the Adenohypophysis of *Myxine glutinosa*', *Z. Zellforsch*, *132*, 451.

Fridberg, G. and Ekengren, B. (1977) 'The Vascularization and the Neuroendocrine Pathways of the Pituitary Gland in the Atlantic Salmon, (*Salmo salar*)', *Can. J. Zool.*, *55*, 1284.

Goos, H.J. Th. (1978) 'Hypophysiotropic Centers in the Brain of Amphibia and Fish', *Am. Zool.*, *18*, 401.

Goos, H.J. Th. and Murathanoglu, O. (1977) 'Localisation of Gonadotropin Releasing Hormone (GRH) in the Forebrain and Neurohypophysis of the Trout (*Salmo gairdneri*), *Cell Tissue Res.*, *181*, 163.

Goossens, N., Dierickx, K. and Vandesande, F. (1977) 'Immunocytochemical Localization of Vasotocin and Isotocin in the Preopticohypophysial Neurosecretory System of Teleosts', *Gen. Comp. Endocrinol.*, *32*, 371.

Green, J.D. (1966) 'The Comparative Anatomy of the Portal Vascular System and of the Innervation of the Hypophysis' in G.W. Harris and B.T. Donovan (eds.) *The Pituitary Gland*, Butterworths, London, p. 127.

Hoar, W.S. (1966) 'Hormonal Activities of the Pars Distalis in Cyclostomes, Fish and Amphibia', in G.W. Harris and B.T. Donovan (eds.), *The Pituitary Gland*, Butterworths, London, p. 242.

Idler, D.R. and Ng, T.B. (1979) 'Studies on Two Types of Gonadotropins from Both Salmon and Carp Pituitaries', *Gen. Comp. Endocrinol.*, *38*, 421.

Kaul, S. and Vollrath, L. (1974) 'The Goldfish Pituitary', *Cell Tissue Res.*, *154*, 211.

Kawauchi, H., Kawazoe, I., Adachi, Y., Buckley, D.I. and Ramachandran, J. (1984) 'Chemical and Biological Characterization of Salmon Melanocyte-stimulating Hormones', *Gen. Comp. Endocrinol.*, *53*, 37.

Kayes, T. (1977) 'Effect of Hypophysectomy, Beef Growth Hormone Replacement Therapy, Pituitary Autotransplantation and Environmental Salinity on Growth in the Black Bullhead (*Ictalurus melas*)', *Gen. Comp. Endocrinol.*, *33*, 371.

Kerr, T. and van Oordt, P.G.W.J. (1966) 'The Pituitary of the African Lungfish (*Protopterus sp.*)', *Gen. Comp. Endocrinol.*, *7*, 549.

Lam, T.J. (1972) 'Prolactin and Hydromineral Regulation in Fishes', *Gen. Comp. Endocrinol.* Suppl. 3, 328.

McKeown, B.A., Jenks, B.G. and van Overbeeke, A.P. (1980) 'Biosynthesis and Release of Prolactin from the Pituitary Gland of the Rainbow Trout, *Salmo gairdneri*, *Comp. Biochem. Physiol.*, *65B*, 705.

Morley, M., Chadwick, A. and El Tounsy, E.M. (1981) 'The Effect of Prolactin on Water Absorption by the Intestine of Trout (*Salmo gairdneri*)', *Gen. Comp. Endocrinol.*, *44*, 6a.

Ng, T.B. and Idler, D. (1980) 'Gonadotropic Regulation of Androgen Production in Flounder and Salmonids', *Gen. Comp. Endocrinol.*, *42*, 25.

Ng, T.B., Idler, D.R. and Eales, J.G. (1982) 'Pituitary Hormones that Stimulate the Thyroidal System in Teleost Fishes', *Gen. Comp. Endocrinol.*, *48*, 372.

Pang, P.K.T. (1977) 'Osmoregulatory Functions of Neurohypophysial Hormones in Fishes and Amphibians', *Am. Zool.*, *17*, 739.

Pang, P.K.T. (1981) 'Pituitary and Prolactin Influences on Calcium Regulation in the Mud Puppy, *Necturus maculosus*', *Gen. Comp. Endocrinol.*, *44*, 524.

Peter, R.E. (1973) 'Neuroendocrinology of Teleosts', *Am. Zool.*, *13*, 743.

Pickford, G.E. and Atz, J.W. (1957) *The Physiology of the Pituitary Gland of Fishes*. New York Zoological Society.

Prunet, P. and Houdebine, L. (1984) 'Purification and Biological Characterization of Chinook Salmon Prolactin', *Gen. Comp. Endocrinol.*, *53*, 49.

Sage, M. and Bern, H.A. (1971) 'Cytophysiology of the Teleost Pituitary', *Int. Rev. Cytol.*, *31*, 339.

Sawyer, W.H. (1966) 'Neurohypophysial Principles of Vertebrates', in G.W. Harris and B.T. Donovan (eds.), *The Pituitary Gland*, Butterworths, London, p. 307.

Schreibman, M.P., Leatherland, J.F. and McKeown, B.A. (1973) 'Functional Morphology of the Teleost Pituitary Gland', *Am. Zool.*, *13*, 719.

van Kemenade, J.A.M. and Kremers, J.W. (1975) 'The Pituitary Gland of the Coelacanth Fish, *Latimeria chalumnae* Smith: General Structure and Adenohypophysial Cell Types', *Cell Tissue Res.*, *163*, 291.

van Oordt, P.G.W.J. (1979) 'A Typology of the Gnathostome Adenohypophysis with Some Emphasis on its Gonadotropic Function', *Basic and Applied Histochemistry*, *23*, 187.

Chapter 2: Thyroid

(a) Thyroid

Brown, C.L., Dashow, L., Epple, A.W. and Stetson, M.H. (1982) 'Thyroid Hormone Clearance Kinetics in Adult Sea Lampreys, *Petromyzon marinus*', *Gen. Comp. Endocrinol.*, *47*, 333.

Brown, S. and Eales, J.G. (1977) 'Measurement of l-thyroxine and 3, 5, 3'-triiodo-l-thyronine Levels in Fish Plasma by Radioimmunoassay', *Can. J. Zool.*, *55*, 293.

Chan. H.H. and Eales, J.G. (1976) 'Influence of Bovine TSH on Plasma Thyroxine Levels and Thyroid Function in Brook Trout, *Salvelinus fontinalis*', *Gen. Comp. Endocrinol.*, *28*, 461.

Chavin, W. (1976) 'The Thyroid of the Sarcopterygian Fishes (Dipnoi and Crossopterygii) and the Origin of the Tetrapod Thyroid', *Gen. Comp. Endocrinol.*, *30*, 142.

Dodd, J.M. and Matty, A.J. (1964) 'Comparative Aspects of Thyroid Function' in R. Pitt-Rivers and W.R. Trotter (eds.) *The Thyroid Gland*, Butterworths, London, Vol. 1, p. 303.

Eales, J.G. (1982) 'Circannual Cycles of Thyroid Hormones in Plasma of Winter Flounder (*Pseudopleuronectes americanus*)', *Can. J. Zool.*, *60*, 304.

Eales, J.G., Chang, J.P., van der Kraak, G., Omeljaniuk, R.J. and Uin, L. (1982) 'Effects of Temperature on Plasma Thyroxine and Iodide Kinetics in Rainbow Trout, *Salmo gairdneri*', *Gen. Comp. Endocrinol.*, *47*, 295.

Eales, J.G., Hughes, M. and Uin, L. (1981) 'Effect of Food Intake on Diet Variation in Plasma Thyroid Hormone Levels in Rainbow Trout, *Salmo gairdneri*', *Gen. Comp. Endocrinol.*, *45*, 167.

Hoar, W.S. (1958) 'Effects of Synthetic Thyroxine and Gonadal Steroids on the Metabolism of Goldfish', *Can. J. Zool.*, *36*, 113.

Hunt, D.W.C. and Eales, J.G. (1979) 'The Influence of Testosterone Proprionate on Thyroid Function of Immature Rainbow Trout, *Salmo gairdneri*', *Gen. Comp. Endocrinol.*, *37*, 115.

Jackson, R.G. and Sage, M. (1973) 'A Comparison of the Effects of Mammalian TSH on the Thyroid Glands of the Teleost *Galeichthys felis* and the Elasmobranch *Dasyatis sabina*', *Comp. Biochem. Physiol.*, *44A*, 867.

Leatherland, J.F. (1982) 'Environmental Physiology of the Teleostean Thyroid Gland: a Review', *Env. Biol. Fish.*, *7*, 83.

Leatherland, J.F. and Sonstegard, R.A. (1981) 'Thyroid Function, Pituitary Structure and Serum Lipids in Great Lakes Coho Salmon, *Oncorhynchus kisutch*, 'Jacks' Compared with Sexually Immature Spring Salmon', *J. Fish Biol.*, *18*, 643.

Lintrop, S.P. and Youson, J.H. (1983) 'Concentration of Triiodothyronine in the Sera of the Sea Lamprey, *Petromyzon marinus*, and the Brook Lamprey, *Lampetra lamottenii*, at Various Phases of the Life Cycle', *Gen. Comp. Endocrinol.*, *49*, 187.

Lintrop, S.P. and Youson, J.H. (1983) 'Binding of Triiodothyronine to Hepatic Nuclei from Sea Lampreys, *Petromyzon marinus*, at Various Stages of the Life Cycle', *Gen. Comp. Endocrinol.*, *49*, 428.

Massey, B.D. and Smith, C.L. (1968) 'The Action of Thyroxine on Mitochondrial Respiration and Phosphorylation in the Trout, *Salmo trutta fario*', *Comp. Biochem. Physiol.*, *25*, 241.

Matty, A.J. (1960) 'Thyroid Cycles in Fish', *Symp. Zool. Soc. London*, *2*, p. 1.

Matty, A.J., Chaudhry, M.A. and Lone, K.P. (1982) 'The Effect of Thyroid Hormones and Temperature on Protein and Nucleic Acid Contents of Liver and Muscle of *Sarotherodon mossambica*', *Gen. Comp. Endocrinol.*, *47*, 497.

Monaco, F., Dominici, R., Andreoli, M., De Pirro, R. and Roche, J. (1981) 'Thyroid Hormone Formation in Thyroglobulin Synthesized in the Amphioxus (*Branchiostoma lanceolatum Pallas*)', *Comp. Biochem. Physiol.*, *70B*, 341.

Paul, A.K. and Medda, A.K. (1983) 'Comparative Study on the Effects of Thyroxine on Protein, RNA and DNA Contents of Liver of Different Vertebrates at Different Stages of Life', *Gegenbaurs morph. Jahrb., Leipzig*, *129*, 239.

Ray, A.K. and Medda, A.K. (1976) 'Effects of Thyroid Hormones and Analogues on Ammonia and Urea Excretion in Lata Fish (*Ophicephalus punctatus*)', *Gen.*

Comp. Endocrinol., 29, 190.

Spieler, R.E. (1979) 'Diel Rhythms of Circulating Prolactin, Cortisol, Thyroxine and Triiodothyronine Levels in Fishes: a Review', *Rev. Can. Biol., 38*, 301.

Spieler, R.E. and Noeske, T.A. (1979) 'Diel Variations in Circulating Levels of Triiodothyronine and Thyroxine in Goldfish, *Carassius auratus*', *Can. J. Zool., 57*, 665.

van der Kraak, G.J. and Eales, J.G. (1980) 'Saturable 3,5,3'-triiodo-1-thyronine-binding Sites in Liver Nuclei of Rainbow Trout (*Salmo gairdneri*)', *Gen. Comp. Endocrinol., 42*, 437.

Waterman, A.J. and Gorbman, A. (1963) 'Thyroid Tissue and Some of its Properties in the Hagfish, *Myxine glutinosa*', *Gen. Comp. Endocrinol., 3*, 58.

Woodhead, A.D. (1966) 'Thyroid Activity in the Ovo-viviparous Elasmobranch *Squalus acanthias*', *J. Zool., 148*, 238.

Wright, G.M. and Youson, J.H. (1980) 'Variations in Serum Levels of Thyroxine in Anadromous Larval Lampreys, *Petromyzon marinus*', *Gen. Comp. Endocrinol., 41*, 321.

(b) Ultimobranchial

McMillan, P.J., Hooker, W.M., Roos, B.A. and Deftos, L.J. (1976) 'Ultimobranchial Gland of the Trout (*Salmo gairdneri*). 1. Immunohisto-chemistry and Radioimmunoassay of Calcitonin', *Gen. Comp. Endocrinol., 28*, 313.

Pang, P.K.T. (1971) 'Calcitonin and Ultimobranchial Glands in Fishes', *J. Exp. Zool., 178*, 89.

van Noorden, S. and Pearse, A.G.E. (1972) 'The Ultimobranchial Gland of the Dogfish, *Scyliorhinus canicula*, Immunofluorescence Cross-reactivities with Anti-sera to Different Calcitonins', *Histochemie, 30*, 97.

Wendelaar Bonga, S.E. (1980) 'Effect of Synthetic Salmon Calcitonin and Low Ambient Calcium on Plasma Calcium, Ultimobranchial Cells, Stannius Bodies, and Prolactin Cells in the Teleost, *Gasterosteus aculeatus*', *Gen. Comp. Endocrinol., 40*, 99.

Chapter 3: Pancreas and Gastrointestinal Hormones

(a) Pancreas

Brinn, J.E. (1973) 'The Pancreatic Islets of Bony Fishes', *Am. Zool., 13*, 653-

Cowey, C.B., Knox, D., Walton, M.J. and Adron, J.W. (1977) 'The Regulation of Gluconeogenesis by Diet and Insulin in Rainbow Trout, (*Salmo gairdneri*)', *Br. J. Nutr., 38*, 463.

Epple, A. and Kocsis, J.J. (1980) 'The Effects of Pancreatectomy on Tissue Taurine under Varying Osmotic and Nutritional Conditions', *Comp. Biochem. Physiol., 65A*, 139.

Epple, A. and Lewis, T.L. (1973) 'Comparative Histophysiology of the Pancreatic Islets', *Am. Zool., 13*, 567.

Epple, A. and Lewis, T.L. (1977) 'Metabolic Effects of Pancreatectomy and Hypophysectomy in the Yellow Eel, *Anguilla rostrata*', *Gen. Comp. Endocrinol., 32*, 294.

Epple, A. and Miller, S.B. (1981) 'Pancreatectomy in the Eel: Osmoregulation Effects', *Gen. Comp. Endocrinol., 45*, 453.

Falkmer, S. and Matty, A.J. (1966) 'Blood Sugar Regulation in the Hagfish, *Myxine Glutinosa*', *Gen. Comp. Endocrinol., 6*, 334.

246 Bibliography

Fletcher, D.J., Noe, B.D., and Hunt, E.L. (1978) 'Studies on Insulin Biosynthesis in the Channel Cafish, (*Ictalurus punctatus*)', *Gen. Comp. Endocrinol., 35,* 127.

Fletcher, D.J., Trent, D.F. and Weir, G.C. (1983) 'Catfish Somatostatin is Unique to Piscine Tissues', *Regulatory Peptides, 5,* 181.

Grant, P.T. and Reid, B.M. (1968) 'Isolation and Partial Amino Acid Sequence of Insulin from the Islet Tissue of Cod, (*Gadus callaris*)', *Biochem. J., 106,* 531.

Hardisty, M.W., Zelnik, P.R. and Moore, I.A. (1975) 'The Effects of Subtotal and Total Isletectomy in the River Lamprey, *Lampetra fluviatilis*', *Gen. Comp. Endocrinol., 27,* 179.

Hardisty, M.W., Zelnik, P.R. and Wright, V.C. (1976) 'The Effects of Hypoxia on Blood Sugar Levels and on the Endocrine Pancreas, Interrenal, and Chromaffin Tissues of the Lamprey, *Lampetra fluivatilis*', *Gen. Comp. Endocrinol., 28,* 184.

Huth, A. and Rapoport, T.A. (1982) 'Regulation of the Biosynthesis of Insulin in Isolated Brockmann bodies of the Carp (*Cyprinus carpio*)', *Gen. Comp. Endocrinol., 46,* 158.

Ince, B.W. (1979) 'Insulin Secretion from the *in situ* Perfused Pancreas of the European Silver Eel, *Anguilla anguilla*', *Gen. Comp. Endocrinol., 37,* 533.

Ince, B.W. (1980) 'Amino Acid Stimulation of Insulin Secretion from the *in situ* Perfused Eel Pancreas: Modification by Somatostatin, Adrenaline, and Theophylline', *Gen. Comp. Endocrinol., 40,* 275.

Ince, B.W. and Thorpe, A. (1977) 'Glucose and Amino Acid-stimulated Insulin Release *in vivo* in the European Silver Eel, (*Anguilla anguilla*)', *Gen. Comp. Endocrinol., 31,* 249.

Ince, B.W. and Thorpe, A. (1977) 'Plasma Insulin and Glucose Responses to Glucagon and Catecholamines in the European Silver Eel, (*Anguilla anguilla*)', *Gen. Comp. Endocrinol., 33,* 453.

Inui, Y. and Yokote, M. (1977) 'Effects of Glucagon on Amino Acid Metabolism in Japanese Eels, *Anguilla japonica*', *Gen. Comp. Endocrinol., 33,* 167.

Inui, Y., Yu. J.Y.-L. and Gorbman, A. (1978) 'Effect of Bovine Insulin on the Incorporation of C-glycine into Protein and Carbohydrate in Liver and Muscle of Hagfish, *Eptatretus stouti*', *Gen. Comp. Endocrinol., 36,* 133.

Klein, C. (1978) 'Use of Immunocytochemical Staining for Correlative Light and Electron Microscopic Investigation of D cells in the Pancreatic Islet of *Xiphophorus helleri*', *Cell Tissue Res. 194,* 399.

Leibson, L. and Plisetskaya, E.M. (1968) 'Effect of Insulin on Blood Sugar Level and Glycogen Content in Organs of Some Cyclostomes and Fish', *Gen. Comp. Endocrinol., 11,* 381.

Leibson, L.G. and Plisetskaya, E.M. (1969) 'Hormonal Control of Blood Sugar Level in Cyclostomes', *Gen. Comp. Endocrinol.,* Suppl. 2, 528.

Lewis, T.L. and Epple, A. (1972) 'Pancreatectomy in the Eel: Effects on Serum Glucose and Cholesterol', *Science, 178,* 1286.

Makower, A., Dettmer, R., Rapaport, T.A., Knospe, S., Behlke, J., Prehn, S., Franke, P., Etzold, G. and Rosenthal, S. (1981) 'Carp Insulin: Amino Acid Sequence, Biological Activity and Structural Properties', *Eur. J. Biochem., 122,* 339.

Muggeo, M., van Obberghen, E., Kahn, C.R., Roth, J., Ginsberg, B.H., De Meyts, P., Emdin, S.O. and Falkmer, S. (1979) 'The Insulin Receptor and Insulin of the Atlantic Hagfish', *Diabetes, 28,* 175.

Ohgawara, H., Tasaka, Y. and Kanazawa, Y. (1978) 'Effect of the Bonito Insulin on the Insulin Release from Monolayer Culture of Rat Pancreas', *Endocrinol. Japan, 25,* 443.

Patent, G.J. (1973) 'The Chondrichthyean Endocrine Pancreas: What are its Functions?' *Am. Zool., 13,* 639.

Steiner, D.F., Peterson, J.D., Tager, H., Emdin, S., Osterberg, Y. and Falkmer, S.

(1973) 'Comparative Aspects of Proinsulin and Insulin Structure and Biosynthesis', *Am. Zool.*, *13*, 591.

Stewart, J.K., Goodner, C.J., Koerker, D.J., Gorbman, A., Ensinck, J. and Kuafman, M. (1978) 'Evidence for a Biological Role of Somatostatin in the Pacific Hagfish, *Eptatretus stouti*', *Gen. Comp. Endocrinol.*, *36*, 408.

Thomas, N.W. (1970) 'Morphology of Endocrine Cells in the Islet Tissue of the Cod, *Gadus callaris*', *Acta Endocrinologica*, *63*, 679.

Trakatellis, A.C., Tada, K., Yamaji, K. and Gardiki-Kouidou, P. (1975) 'Isolation and Partial Characterization of Anglerfish Proglucogon', *Biochemistry*, *14*, 1508.

Wagner, G.F. and McKeown, B.A. (1981) 'Immunocytochemical Localisation of Hormone-producing Cells within the Pancreatic Islets of the Rainbow Trout, (*Salmo gairdneri*)', *Cell Tissue Res.*, *221*, 181.

(b) Gastrointestinal Hormones

Barrington, E.J.W. and Dockray, G.J. (1972) 'Cholecystokinin-pancreozymin-like Activity in the Eel, (*Anguilla anguilla*)', *Gen. Comp. Endocrinol.*, *19*, 80.

Dockray, G.J. (1978) 'Comparative Biochemistry and Physiology of Gut Hormones', *Ann. Rev. Physiol.*, *41*, 83.

Holmgren, S., Vaillant, C. and Dimaline, R. (1982) 'VIP-, Substance P-, Gastrin/ CCK-, Bombesin-, Somatostatin- and Glucagon-like Immunoreactivities in the Gut of the Rainbow Trout, *Salmo gairdneri*', *Cell Tissue Res.*, *223*, 141.

Holmquist, A.L., Dockray, G.J., Rosenquist, G.L. and Walsh, J.H. (1979) 'Immunochemical Characterization of Cholecystokinin-like Peptides in Lamprey Gut and Brain', *Gen. Comp. Endocrinol.*, *37*, 474.

Holstein, B. and Humphrey, C.S. (1980) 'Stimulation of Gastric Acid Secretion and Suppression of VIP-like Immunoreactivity by Bombesin in the Atlantic Codfish, *Gadus morhua*', *Acta Physiol. Scand.*, *109*, 217.

Johnson, D.A., Noe, B.D. and Bauer, G.E. (1982) 'Pancreatic Polypeptide (PP)- like Immunoreactivity in the Pancreatic Islets of the Anglerfish (*Lophius americanus*) and the Channel Catfish (*Ictalurus punctatus*)', *Anat. Rec.*, *204*, 61.

van Noorden, S. and Falkmer, S. (1980) 'Gut-islet Endocrinology — Some Evolutionary Aspects', *Invest. Cell. Pathol.*, *3*, 21.

van Noorden, S., Greenberg, J. and Pearse, A.G.E. (1972) 'Cytochemical and Immunofluorescence Investigations on Polypeptide Hormone Localisation in the Pancreas and Gut of the Larval Lamprey', *Gen. Comp. Endocrinol.*, *19*, 192.

Vigna, S.R. and Gorbman, A. (1977) 'Effects of Cholecystokinin, Gastrin, and Related Peptides on Coho Salmon Gallbladder Contraction *in vitro*', *Am. J. Physiol.*, *232*, E485.

Chapter 4: The 'Adrenal' and the Kidney Hormones

(a) Chromaffin Tissue

Abrahamsson, T. (1979) 'Phenylethanolamine-N-methyl Transferase Activity and Catecholamine Storage and Release from Chromaffin Tissue of the Spiny Dogfish, *Squalus acanthias*', *Comp. Biochem. Physiol.*, *64C*, 169.

Abrahamsson, T., Johnsson, T. and Nilsson, S. (1979) 'Catecholamine Synthesis in the Chromaffin Tissue of the African Lungfish, *Protopterus aethiopicus*', *Acta Physiol. Scand.*, *107*, 149.

248   *Bibliography*

Butler, P.J., Taylor, E.W., Capra, M.F. and Davidson, W. (1979) 'The Effect of Hypoxia on the Levels of Circulating Catecholamines in the Dogfish, *Scyliorhinus canicula*', *J. Comp. Physiol.*, *127*, 325.

Coupland, R.E. (1979) 'Catecholamines' in E.J.W. Barrington (ed.), *Hormones and Evolution*, Academic Press, London, Vol. 1, p. 309.

deRoos, R. and deRoos, C.C. (1972) 'Comparative Effects of the Pituitary-adrenocortical Axis and Catecholamines on Carbohydrate Metabolism in Elasmobranch Fish', *Gen. Comp. Endocrinol., Suppl. 3*, 192.

deRoos, R. and deRoos, C.C. (1978) 'Elevation of Plasma Glucose Levels by Catecholamines in Elasmobranch Fish', *Gen. Comp. Endocrinol.*, *34*, 447.

Epple, A., Vogel, W.H. and Nibbio, B.J. (1982) 'Catecholamines in Head and Body Blood of Eels and Rats', *Comp. Biochem. Physiol.*, *71C*, 115.

Forster, M.E. (1981) 'Effects of Catecholamines on the Hearts and Ventral Aortas of the Eels, *Anguilla australis Scmidtii* and *Anguilla dieffenbachii*', *Comp. Biochem. Physiol.*, *70C*, 85.

Jonsson, A.-C., Wahlqvist, I. and Hansson, T. (1983) 'Effects of Hypophysectomy and Cortisol on the Catecholamine Biosynthesis and Catecholamine Content in Chromaffin Tissue from the Rainbow Trout, *Salmo gairdneri*', *Gen. Comp. Endocrinol.*, *51*, 278.

Larsson, A.L. (1973) 'Metabolic Effects of Epinephrine and Norepinephrine in the Eel, *Anguilla anguilla*', *Gen. Comp. Endocrinol.*, *20*, 115.

Le Bras, Y.M. (1982) 'Effects of Anaesthesia and Surgery on Levels of Adrenaline and Noradrenaline in the Blood Plasma of the Eel (*Anguilla anguilla*), *Comp. Biochem. Physiol.*, *72C*, 141.

Mazeaud, M.M. and Mazeaud, F. (1981) 'Adrenergic Responses to Stress in Fish' in A.D. Pickering (ed.), *Stress in Fish*, Academic Press, London, p. 49.

Oguri, M. (1960) 'Studies of the Adrenal Glands of Teleosts-3. On the Distribution of Chromaffin Cells and Interrenal Cells in the Head Kidney of Fishes', *Bull. Jap. Soc. Scient. Fish*, *26*, 443.

Ostlund, E. and Fange, R. (1962) 'Vasodilation by Adrenaline and Noradrenaline, and the Effects of Some Other Substances on Perfused Fish Gills', *Comp. Biochem. Physiol.*, *5*, 307.

Pic, P., Mayer-Gostan, N. and Maetz, J. (1975) 'Branchial Effects of Epinephrine in the Seawater Adapted Mullet. 2, Na and Cl Extrusion', *Am. J. Physiol.*, *228*, 441.

Tuurala, H., Soivio, A. and Nikinmaa, M. (1982) 'The Effect of Adrenaline on Heart Rate and Blood Pressure in *Salmo gairdneri* at Two Temperatures', *Ann. Zool. Fennici*, *19*, 47.

Umminger, B.L., Benziger, D. and Levy, L. (1975) 'In Vitro Stimulation of Hepatic Glycogen Phosphorylase Activity by Epinephrine and Glucagon in the Killifish, *Fundulus heteroclitus*', *Comp. Biochem. Physiol.*, *51C*, 111.

Von Euler, U.S. and Fange, R. (1961) 'Catecholamines in Nerves and Organs of *Myxine glutinosa*, *Squalus acanthias* and *Gadus callarias*', *Gen. Comp. Endocrinol.*, *1*, 191.

(b) Interrenal Tissue

Assem, H. and Hanke, W. (1981) 'Cortisol and Osmotic Adjustment of the Euryhaline Teleost, *Sarotherodon mossambicus*', *Gen. Comp. Endocrinol.*, *43*, 370.

Bhattacharyya, T.P., Butler, D.G. and Youson, J.H. (1981) 'Distribution and Structure of the Adrenocortical Homologue in the Garpike', *Am. J. Anat.*, *160*, 246.

Bry, C. (1982) 'Daily Variations in Plasma Cortisol Levels of Individual Female

Rainbow Trout, *Salmo gairdneri*: Evidence for a Post-feeding Peak in Well-adapted Fish', *Gen. Comp. Endocrinol.*, *48*, 462.

Butler, D.G. (1973) 'Structure and Function of Adrenal Gland of Fishes', *Am. Zool.*, *13*, 839.

Buus, D. and Larsen, L.O. (1975) 'Absence of Known Corticosteroids in Blood of River Lampreys (*Lampetra fluviatilis*) after Treatment with Mammalian Corticotropin', *Gen. Comp. Endocrinol.*, *26*, 96.

Chan, D.K.O. and Woo, N.Y.S. (1978) 'Effect of Cortisol on the Metabolism of the Eel, *Anguilla japonica*', *Gen. Comp. Endocrinol.*, *35*, 205.

Chavin, W. and Olivereau, M. (1961) 'Adrenal Histochemistry of Fresh Water and Marine Teleosts', *Am. Zool.*, *1*, 204

Chester Jones, I. (1975) *The Adrenal Cortex*, Cambridge University Press.

Chester Jones, I. and Henderson, I.W. (eds.) (1980) *General, Comparative and Clinical Endocrinology of the Adrenal Cortex*, Vols. 1-3, Academic Press, London.

deRoos, R. and deRoos, C.C. (1972) 'Elevation of Plasma Glucose Levels by Mammalian ACTH in the Spiny Dogfish Shark (*Squalus acanthias*)', *Gen. Comp. Endocrinol.*, *21*, 403.

Holmes, W.N., Phillips, J.G. and Chester Jones, I. (1963) 'Adrenocortical Factors Associated with Adaptation of Vertebrates to Marine Environments', in *Recent Progress in Hormone Research*, Academic Press, New York, Vol. 10, p. 619.

Idler, D.R. and Kane, K.M. (1980) 'Cytosol Receptor Glycoprotein for 1α-Hydroxycorticosterone in Tissues of an Elasmobranch Fish (*Raja ocellata*)', *Gen. Comp. Endocrinol.*, *42*, 259.

Idler, D.R. and Truscott, B. (1972) 'Corticosteroids in Fish' in D.R. Idler (ed.), *Steroids in Non-mammalian Vertebrates*, Academic Press, London, p. 127.

Leach, G.J. and Taylor, M.H. (1980) 'The Role of Cortisol in Stress-induced Metabolic Changes in *Fundulus heteroclitus*', *Gen. Comp. Endocrinol.*, *42*, 219.

Mainoya, J.R. (1982) 'Water and NaCl Absorption by the Intestine of the Tilapia *Sarotherodon mossambicus* Adapted to Fresh Water or Seawater and the Possible Role of Prolactin and Cortisol', *J. Comp. Physiol.*, *146*, 1.

Nandi, J. (1962) 'The Structure of the Interrenal Gland in Fishes', *Univ. of Calif. Publs. Zool.*, *65*, 129.

Pickering, A.D. (ed.) *Stress and Fish*, Academic Press, London.

Pickering, A.D. and Pottinger, T.G. (1983) 'Seasonal and Diel Changes in Plasma Cortisol Levels of the Brown Trout, *Salmo trutta*', *Gen. Comp. Endocrinol.*, *49*, 232.

Sangerlang, G.B., Freeman, H.C., Fleming, R.B. and McMenemy, M. (1980) 'The Determination of Cortisol in Fish Plasma by Radioimmunoassay', *Gen. Comp. Endocrinol.*, *40*, 459.

Truscott, B. (1979) 'Steroid Metabolism in Fish. Identification of Steroid Moieties of Hydrolyzable Conjugates of Cortisol in the Bile of Trout, *Salmo gairdneri*', *Gen. Comp. Endocrinol.*, *38*, 196.

Weisbart, M. and Jenkins, D.K. (1981) 'Radioimmunoassay of Cortisol in the Adult Atlantic Salmon, *Salmo salar*', *Gen. Comp. Endocrinol.*, *43*, 364.

(c) Renin-Angiotensin System

Bailey, J.R. and Fenwick, J.C. (1974) 'Effect of Angiotensin II and Corpuscle of Stannius Extract on Total and Ionic Plasma Levels and Blood Pressure in Intact Eels (*Anguilla rostrata*)', *Can. J. Zool.*, *53*, 630.

Bailey, J.R. and D.J. Randall (1981) 'Renal Perfusion-pressure and Renin Secretion in the Rainbow Trout, *Salmo gairdneri*', *Can. J. Zool.*, *59*, 1220.

250   *Bibliography*

Brown, J.A., Oliver, J.A. and Henderson, I.W. (1980) 'Angiotensin and Single Nephron Glomerular Function in the Trout, *Salmo gairdneri*', *Am. J. Physiol.*, *239*, R509.
Capelli, J.P., Wesson, L.G. and Aponte, G.E. (1970) 'A Phylogenetic Study of the Renin-angiotensin System', *Am. J. Physiol.*, *218*, 1171.
Fenwick, J.C. and So, Y.P. (1981) 'Effect of an Angiotensin on the Net Influx of Calcium across an Isolated Perfused Eel Gill', *Can. J. Zool.*, *59*, 119.
Malvin, R.L. and Vander, A.J. (1967) 'Plasma Renin Activity in Marine Teleosts and Cetacea', *Am. J. Physiol.*, *213*, 1582.
Nishimura, H., Croften, J.T., Norton, V.M. and Share, L. (1977) 'Angiotensin Generation in Teleost Fish Determined by Radioimmunoassay and Bioassay', *Gen. Comp. Endocrinol.*, *32*, 236.
Nishimura, H., Ogwana, M. and Sawyer, W.H. (1973) 'Renin-angiotensin System in Primitive Bony Fishes and a Holocephalian', *Am. J. Physiol.*, *224*, 950.
Pang, P.K.T., Pang, R.K., Liu, V.K.Y. and Sokabe, H. (1981) 'Effect of Fish Angiotensins and Angiotensin-like Substances on Killifish Calcium Regulation', *Gen. Comp. Endocrinol.*, *43*, 292.
Sokabe, H. and Ogawa, M. (1974) 'Comparative Studies of the Juxtaglomerular Apparatus', *Int. Rev. Cytol.*, *37*, 271.
Sokabe, H., Oide, H., Ogawa, M. and Utida, S. (1973) 'Plasma Renin Activity in Japanese Eels (*Anguilla japonica*) Adapted to Seawater or in Dehydration', *Gen. Comp. Endocrinol.*, *21*, 160.
Takemoto, Y., Nakajma, T., Hasegawa, Y., Watanabe, T.X., Sokabe, H., Kumagae, S. and Sakakibara, S. (1983) 'Chemical Structures of Angiotensins Formed by Incubating Plasma with the Kidney and Corpuscles of Stannius in the Chum Salmon, *Oncorhynchus*', *Gen. Comp. Endocrinol.*, *51*, 219.
Taylor, A.A. (1977) 'Comparative Physiology of the Renin-angiotensin System', *Fed. Proc.*, *36*, 1776.

Chaper 5: Gonadal Hormones

Baggerman, B. (1968) 'Hormonal Control of Reproductive and Parental Behaviour in Fishes' in E.J.W. Barrington and C. Barker Jorgensen (eds.), *Perspectives in Endocrinology*, Academic Press, London, p. 351.
Baggerman, B. (1980) 'Photoperiodic and Endogenous Control of the Annual Reproductive Cycle in Teleost Fishes' in M.A. Ali (ed.), *Environmental Physiology of Fishes*, Plenum, New York, p. 533.
Bern, H.A. and Chieffi, G. (1968) 'Bibliography on the Steroid Hormones of Fishes', *Publ. Staz. Zool. Napoli*, *36*, 287.
Chang, Y. and Huang, F. (1982) 'The Mode of Action of Carp Gonadotropin on the Stimulation of Androgen Production by Carp Testis *in vitro*', *Gen. Comp. Endocrinol.*, *48*, 147.
Demski, L.S. and Hornby, P.J. (1982) 'Hormonal Control of Fish Reproductive Behavior: Brain-Gonadal Steroid Interactions', *Can. J. Fish. Aquat. Sci.*, *39*, 36.
Dodd, J.M. (1964) 'Endocrine Patterns in the Reproduction of Lower Vertebrates', *Excerpta Medica Int. Congress Series*, *83*, 124.
Dodd, J.M. (1975) 'The Hormones of Sex and Reproduction and Their Effects in Fish and Lower Chordates: Twenty Years on', *Am. Zool.* (Suppl. 1), *15*, 137.
Dodd, J.M., Evenett, P.J. and Goddard, C.K. (1960) *Symp. Zool. Soc. London*, *1*, 77.

Forbes, T.R. (1961) 'Endocrinology of Reproduction in Cold-blooded Vertebrates' in W.C. Young and G.W. Corner (eds.), *Sex and Internal Secretions*, Williams and Wilkins, Baltimore, Vol. II, p. 1035.

Gielen, J. Th. and Goos, H.J.Th. (1983) 'The Brain-pituitary-gonadal Axis in the Rainbow Trout, *Salmo gairdneri*', *Cell. Tissue Res., 233*, 377.

Hardisty, M.W. (1965) 'Sex Differentiation and Gonadogenesis in Lampreys', *J. Zool., 146*, 345.

Hoar, W.S. (1965) 'Comparative Physiology: Hormones and Reproduction in Fishes', *Ann. Rev. Physiol., 27*, 51.

Idler, D.R. (1979) 'Quantification of Vitellogenin in Atlantic Salmon (*Salmo salar*) Plasma by Radioimmunoassay; *J. Fish. Res. Board Can., 36*, 574.

Katz. Y., Dashow, L. and Epple, A. (1982) 'Circulating Steroid Hormones of Anadromous Sea Lampreys under Various Experimental Conditions', *Gen. Comp. Endocrinol., 48*, 261.

Kime, D.E. (1980) 'Comparative Aspects of Testicular Androgen Biosynthesis in Nonmammalian Vertebrates' in G. Delrio and J. Brachet (eds.) *Steroids and Their Mechanism of Action in Nonmammalian Vertebrates*, Raven Press, New York.

Kime, D.E. and Rafter, J.J. (1981) 'Biosynthesis of 15-hydroxylated Steroids by Gonads of the River Lamprey, *Lampetra fluviatilis, in vitro*', *Gen. Comp. Endocrinol., 44*, 69.

Lambert, J.G.D. (1970) 'The Ovary of the Guppy, *Poecilia reticulata*', *Gen. Comp. Endocrinol., 15*, 464.

Larsen, L.O. (1980) 'Physiology of Adult Lampreys, with Special Regard to Natural Starvation, Reproduction, and Death after Spawning', *Can. J. Fish. Aquat. Sci., 37*, 1762.

Larsen, L.O. (1982) 'The Role of Hormones in Control of Reproduction in Vertebrates: Case Stories and Generalizations' in A.D.F. Addink and N. Spronk (eds.) *Exogenous and Endogenous Influences on Metabolic and Neural Control*, Pergamon, Oxford, p. 153.

Liley, N.R. (1968) 'The Endocrine Control of Reproductive Behaviour in the Female Guppy, *Poecilia reticulata* Peters', *Anim. Behav., 16*, 318.

Marshall, A.J. (1960) 'Reproduction in Male Bony Fish', *Symp. Zool. Soc. Lond., 1*, 137.

Medda, A.K., Dasmahapatra, A.K. and Ray, A.K. (1980) 'Effect of Oestrogen and Testosterone on the Protein and Nucleic Acid Contents of Liver, Muscle, and Gonad and Plasma Protein Content of Male and Female (Vitellogenic and Nonvitellogenic) Singi Fish, *Heteropneustes fossilis* Boch', *Gen. Comp. Endocrinol., 42*, 427.

Mugiya, Y. (1978) 'Effects of Estradiol-17β on Bone and Otolith Calcification in the Goldfish, *Carassius auratus*', *Bull. Jap. Soc. Sci. Fish., 44*, 1217.

Mugiya, Y. and Ichii, T. (1981) 'Effect of Estradiol-17β on Branchial and Intestinal Calcium Uptake in the Rainbow Trout, *Salmo gairdneri*', *Comp. Biochem. Physiol., 70A*, 97.

Nagahama, Y., Clarke, W.C. and Hoar, W.S. (1978) 'Ultrastructure of Putative Steroid-producing Cells in the Gonads of Coho (*Oncorhynchus kisutch*) and Pink Salmon (*Oncorhynchus gorbuscha*)', *Can. J. Zool., 56*, 2508.

Nagahama, Y., Kagawa, H., and Young, G. (1982) 'Cellular Sources of Sex Steroids in Teleost Gonads', *Can. J. Fish. Aquat. Sci., 39*, 56.

Olivereau, M. (1977) 'Donnees recentes sur le controle endocrinien de la reproduction chez les Teleosteens', *Investigacion Pesquera, 41*, 69.

Ozon, R. (1972) 'Androgens in Fishes, Amphibians, Reptiles and Birds' in D.R. Idler (ed.) *Steroids in Nonmammalian Vertebrates*, Academic Press, London, p. 329.

Ozon, R. (1972) 'Estrogens in Fishes, Amphibians, Reptiles, and Birds' in D.R. Idler (ed.) *Steroids in Nonmammalian Vertebrates*, Academic Press, London, p. 390.

Peter, R.E. (1982) 'Neuroendocrine Control of Reproduction in Teleosts', *Can. J. Fish. Aquat. Sci.*, *39*, 48.

Peter, R.E. and Crim, L.W. (1979) 'Reproductive Endocrinology of Fishes: Gonadal Cycles and Gonadotropin in Teleosts', *Ann. Rev. Physiol.*, *41*, 323.

Pickering, A.D. (1976) 'Effects of Gonadectomy, Oestradiol and Testosterone on the Migrating River Lamprey, *Lampetra fluviatilis*', *Gen. Comp. Endocrinol.*, *28*, 473.

Richter, C.J. and Goos, H.J.Th. (comp.) (1982) *Proceedings of the International Symposium on Reproductive Physiology of Fish*, Pudoc, Wageningen.

Schlaghecke, R. (1983) 'Binding of J-hCG to Rainbow Trout (*Salmo gairdneri*) Testis *in vitro*', *Gen. Comp. Endocrinol.*, *49*, 261.

Scott, A.P., Sumptner, J.P. and Hardiman, P.A. (1983) 'Hormone Changes During Ovulation in the Rainbow Trout (*Salmo gairdneri* Richardson)', *Gen. Comp. Endocrinol.*, *49*, 128.

Soivio, A., Pesonen, S., Teravainen, T., Nakari, T. and Mwensi, R. (1982) 'Seasonal Variations in Oestrogen and Testosterone Levels in the Plasma of Brown Trout (*Salmo trutta lacustris*) and in the Metabolism of Testosterone in its Skin', *Ann. Zool. Fennici*, *19*, 53.

Stacey, N.E. (1981) 'Hormonal Regulation of Female Reproductive Behavior in Fish', *Am. Zool.*, *21*, 305.

Sumpter, J.P., Follett, B.K., Jenkins, N. and Dodd, J.M. (1978) 'Studies on the Purification and Properties of Gonadotrophin from Ventral Lobes of the Pituitary Gland of the Dogfish (*Scyliorhinus canicula*)', *Gen. Comp. Endocrinol.*, *36*, 264.

Turner, R.T., Dickhoff, W.W. and Gorbman, A. (1981) 'Estrogen Binding to *Hepatic Nuclei of Pacific Hagfish, Eptatretus stouti*, *Gen. Comp. Endocrinol.*, *45*, 26.

van den Hurk, R., Lambert, J.G.D. and Peute, J. (1982) :Steroidogenesis in the Gonads of Rainbow Trout Fry (*Salmo gairdneri*) before and after the Onset of Gonadal Sex Differentiation', *Reprod. Nutr. Develop.*, *22*, 413.

van den Hurk, R. and Peute, J. (1979) 'Cyclic Changes in the Ovary of the Rainbow Trout, *Salmo gairdneri*, with Special Reference to Sites of Steroidogenesis', *Cell Tissue Res.*, *199*, 289.

van den Hurk, R., Vermeij, J.A.J., Stegenga, J., Peute, J. and Van Oordt, P.G.W.J. (1978) 'Cyclic Changes in the Testis and Vas Deferens of the Rainbow Trout (*Salmo gairdneri*) with Special Reference to Sites of Steroidogenesis', *Ann. Biol. Anim. Bioch. Biophys.*, *18*, 899.

Weigand, D.M. and Peter, R.E. (1980) 'Effects of Testosterone, Oestradiol-17β and Fasting on Plasma Free Fatty Acids in the Goldfish, *Carassius auratus*', *Comp. Biochem. Physiol.*, *66A*, 323.

Weisbart, M. and Youson, J.H. (1975) 'Steroid Formation in the Larval and Parasitic Adult Sea Lamprey, *Petromyzon marinus*', *Gen. Comp. Endocrinol.*, *27*, 517.

Weisbart, M., Dickhoff, W.W., Gorbman, A. and Idler, D.R. (1980) 'The Presence of Steroids in the Sera of the Pacific Hagfish, *Eptatretus stouti* and the Sea Lamprey, *Petromyzon marinus*', *Gen. Comp. Endocrinol.*, *41*, 506.

Young, G., Crim, L.W., Kagawa, H., Kambegawa, A. and Nagahama, Y. (1983) 'Plasma 17α, 20β-dihydroxy-4-pregnen-3-one Levels During Sexual Maturation of Amago Salmon (*Oncorhynchus rhodurus*): Correlation with Plasma Gonadotropin and *in vitro* Production by Ovarian Follicles', *Gen. Comp. Endocrinol.*, *51*, 96.

Light, and Continuous Darkness on Metamorphosis of Anadromous Sea Lampreys (*Petromyzon marinus*)', *J. exp. Zool.*, *218*, 397.

Delahunty, G., Baoer, G., Prack, M. and de Vlaming, V. (1978) 'Effects of Pinealectomy and Melatonin Treatment on Liver and Plasma Metabolites in the Goldfish, *Carassius auratus*', *Gen. Comp. Endocrinol.*, *35*, 99.

Goudie, C.A., Davis, K.B. and Simco, B.A. (1983) 'Influence of the Eyes and Pineal Gland on Locomotor Activity Patterns of Channel Catfish, *Ictalurus punctatus*', *Physiol. Zool.*, *56*, 10.

Hafeez, M.A. and Quay, W.B. (1970) 'Pineal Acetylserotonin Methyltransferase Activity in the Teleost Fishes, *Hesperoleucus symmetricus* and *Salmo gairdneri* with Evidence for Lack of Effect of Constant Light and Darkness', *Comp. Gen. Pharmacol.*, *1*, 257.

Herwig, H.J. (1976) 'Comparative Ultrastructural Investigations of the Pineal Organ of the Blind Cave Fish, *Anoptichthys jordani*', and its Ancestor, the Eyed River Fish, *Astyanax mexicanus*', *Cell Tissue Res.*, *167*, 297.

Hontela, A. and Peter, R.E. (1980) 'Effects of Pinealectomy, Blinding and Sexual Condition on Serum Gonadotropin Levels in the Goldfish', *Gen. Comp. Endocrinol.*, *40*, 168.

Joss, J. (1973) 'The Pineal Complex, Melatonin, and Color Change in the Lamprey *Lampetra*', *Gen. Comp. Endocrinol.*, *21*, 188.

Kavaliers, M., Firth, B.T. and Ralph, C.L. (1980) 'Pineal Control of the Circadian Rhythm of Colour Change in the Killifish (*Fundulus heteroclitus*)', *Can. J. Zool.*, *58*, 456.

Matty, A.J. (1978) 'Pineal and Some Pituitary Hormone Rhythms in Fish' in J. Thorpe (ed.), *Rhythmic Activity of Fishes*, Academic Press, London, p. 21.

Owens, D.W., Gern, W.A., Ralph, C.L. and Boardman, T.J. (1978) 'Nonrelationship between Plasma Melatonin and Background Adaptation in the Rainbow Trout, *Salmo gairdneri*', *Gen. Comp. Endocrinol.*, *34*, 459.

Reed, B.L. (1968) 'The Control of Circadian Pigment Changes in the Pencil Fish: a Proposed Role for Melatonin', *Life Sci.*, *7*, 961.

Rudeberg, C. (1969) 'Light and Electron Microscopic Studies on the Pineal Organ of the Dogfish, *Scyliorhinus canicula*', *Z. Zellforsh.* *96*, 548.

Rudeberg, C. (1971) 'Structure of the Pineal Organs of *Anguilla anguilla* and *Lebistes reticulatus*', *Z. Zellforsh.*, *122*, 227.

Saxena, P.K. and Anand, K. (1977) 'A Comparison of Ovarian Recrudescence in the Catfish, *Mystus tengara* (*Ham.*), Exposed to Short Photoperiods, to Long Photoperiods, and to Melatonin', *Gen. Comp. Endocrinol.*, *33*, 506.

Smith, J.R. and Lavern, J.W. (1976) 'Alterations in Diurnal Pineal Hydroxyindole-O-methyltransferase (HIOMT) Activity in Steelhead Trout (*Salmo gairdneri*) Associated with Changes in Environmental Background Color', *Comp. Biochem. Physiol.*, *53C*, 33.

Smith, J.R. and Lavern, J. (1976) 'The Regulation of Day-night Changes in Hydroxyindole-O-methyltransferase Activity in the Pineal Gland of Steelhead Trout (*Salmo gairdneri*)', *Can. J. Zool.*, *54*, 1530.

Vivien-Roels, B. and Meiniel, A. (1983) 'Seasonal Variations of Serotonin Content in the Pineal Complex and the Lateral Eye of *Lampetra planeri*', *Gen. Comp. Endocrinol.*, *50*, 323.

Chapter 7: Pheromones

Brett, B.L.H. and Grosse, D.J. (1982) 'A Reproductive Pheromone in the Mexican Poeciliid Fish, *Poecilia chica*', *Copeia* (1), 219.

Colombo, L., Belvedere, P.C., Marconato, A. and Bentivegna, F. (1982) 'Pheromones in Teleost Fish' in C.J.J. Richter and H.J.Th. Goos (comp.), *Proceedings of the International Symposium on Reproductive Physiology of Fish*, Pudoc, Wageningen, p. 84.

Cooper, J.C., Scholz, A.T., Horrall, R.M., Hasler, A.D. and Madison, D.M. (1976) 'Experimental Confirmation of the Olfactory Hypothesis with Artificially Imprinted Homing Coho Salmon (*Oncorhynchus kisutch*)', *J. Fish. Res. Board Can.*, *33*, 703.

Crow, R.T. and Liley, N.R. (1979) 'A Sexual Pheromone in the Guppy, *Poecilia reticulata* (Peters)', *Can. J. Zool.*, *57*, 184.

Doving, K.B., Selset, R. and Thommesen, G. (1980) 'Olfactory Sensitivity to Bile Acids in Salmonid Fishes', *Acta Physiol. Scand.*, *108*, 123.

Fisknes, B. and Doving, K.B. (1982) 'Olfactory Sensitivity to Group-specific Substances in Atlantic Salmon (*Salmo salar*)', *J. Chemical Ecology*, *8*, 1083.

Groves, A.B., Collins, G.B. and Trefetren, G.B. (1968) 'Role of Olfaction and Vision in Choice of Spawning Site by Homing Adult Chinook Salmon, *Oncorhynchus tshawytscha*', *J. Fish Res. Board Can.*, *25*, 867.

Hasler, A.D., Scholz, A.T. and Horrall, R.M. (1978) 'Olfactory Imprinting and Homing in Salmon', *Am. Scientist*, *66*, 347.

Hasler, A.D. and Wisby, W.J. (1951) 'Discrimination of Stream Odors by Fishes and Relation to Parent Stream Behavior', *Am. Naturalist*, *85*, 223.

Honda, H. (1980) 'Female Sex Pheromone of Rainbow Trout, *Salmo gairdneri*, Involved in Courtship Behaviour', *Bull. Jap. soc. Sci. Fish*, *46*, 1109.

Honda, H. (1981) 'On the Female Sex Pheromones and Courtship Behaviour in the Salmonids, *Oncorhynchus masou* and *O. rhodurus*', *Bull Jap. soc. Sci. Fish*, *48*, 47.

Liley, N.R. (1982) 'Chemical Communication in Fish', *Can. J. Fish. Aquat. Sci.*, *39*, 22.

Mackie, A.M. (1975) 'Chemoreception' in D.C. Malins and J.R. Sargent (eds.) *Biochemical and Biophysical Perspectives in Marine Biology*, Vol. 2. Academic Press, London.

Nordeng, H. (1977) 'A Pheromone Hypothesis for Homeward Migration in Anadromous Salmonids', *Oikos*, *28*, 155.

Partridge, B.L., Liley, N.R. and Stacey, N. (1976) 'The Role of Pheromones in the Sexual Behaviour of the Goldfish', *Anim. Behav.*, *24*, 291.

Reutter, K. and Pfeiffer, W. (1973) 'Fluoreszenzmikroskopischer nachweis des schreckstoffes in den schreckstoffzellen der elritze, *Phoxinus phoxinus*', *J. Comp. Physiol.*, *82*, 411.

Selset, R. and Doving, K.B. (1980) 'Behaviour of Mature Anadromous Char (*Salmo alpinus* L.), towards Odorants Produced by Smolts of Their Own Population', *Acta Physiol. Scand.*, *108*, 113.

Solomon, D.J. (1977) 'A Review of Chemical Communication in Freshwater Fish', *J. Fish Biol.*, *11*, 363.

Chapter 8: Migration and Sea-Ranching

Aida, K., Nishioka, R.S. and Bern, H.A. (1980) 'Changes in the Corpuscles of Stannius of Coho Salmon (*Oncorhynchus kisutch*) during Smoltification and Seawater Adaptation', *Gen. Comp. Endocrinol.*, *41*, 296.

Baggerman, B. (1960) 'Salinity Preference, Thyroid Activity and the Seaward Migration of Four Species of Pacific Salmon (*Oncorhynchus*)', *J. Fish Res. Board Can.*, *17*, 295.

Baggerman, B. (1960) 'Factors in the Diadromous Migrations of Fish', *Symp. Zool. Soc. Lond.*, *1*, 33.

Biddiscombe, S. and Idler, D.R. (1983) 'Plasma Levels of Thyroid Hormones in Sockeye Salmon (*Oncorhynchus nerka*) Decrease before Spawning', *Gen. Comp. Endocrinol.*, *52*, 467.

Eales, J.G. (1963) 'A Comparative Study of Thyroid Function in Migrant Juvenile Salmon', *Can. J. Zool.*, *41*, 811.

Folmar, L.C. and Dickoff, W.W. (1979) 'Plasma Thyroxine and Gill Na-K ATPase Changes during Seawater Acclimation of Coho Salmon, *Oncorhynchus kisutch*', *Comp. Biochem. Physiol.*, *63A*, 329.

Folmar, L.C. and Dickhoff, W.W. (1980) 'The Parr-smolt Transformation (Smoltification) and Seawater Adaptation in Salmonids: a Review of Selected Literature', *Aquaculture, 21*, 1.

French, C.J., Hochachka, P.W. and Mommsen, T.P. (1983) 'Metabolic Organisation of Liver during Spawning Migration of Sockeye Salmon', *Am. J. Physiol.*, *245*, R827.

Grau, E.G., Specker, J.L., Nishioka, S. and Bern, H.A. (1982) 'Factors Determining the Occurrence of the Surge in Thyroid Activity in Salmon during Smoltification', *Aquaculture, 28*, 49.

Harden Jones, F.R. (1968) *Fish Migration*, Edward Arnold, London.

Hasler, A.D. (1966) *Underwater Guideposts*, University of Wisconsin Press, Madison.

Hoar, W.S. (1976) 'Smolt Transformation: Evolution Behaviour and Physiology', *J. Fish. Res. Board Can.*, *33*, 1234.

Johansson, N. (1981) 'General Problems in Atlantic Salmon Rearing in Sweden', *Ecol. Bull. (Stockholm)*, *34*, 75.

Johnson, D.W. (1973) 'Endocrine Control of Hydromineral Balance in Teleosts', *Am. Zool.*, *13*, 799.

Koch, H.J.A. (1968) 'Migration' in E.J.W. Barrington and C. Barker Jorgensen (eds.), *Perspectives in Endocrinology*, Academic Press, London, p. 305.

Langdon, J.S., Thorpe, J.E. and Roberts, R.J. (1984) 'Effects of Cortisol and ACTH on Gill Na/K-ATPase, SDH and Chloride Cells in Juvenile Atlantic Salmon, *Salmo salar*', *Comp. Biochem. Physiol.*, *77A*, 9.

Lindahl, K., Lundqvist, H. and Rydevik, M. (1983) 'Plasma Thyroxine Levels and Thyroid Gland Histology in Baltic Salmon (*Salmo salar L.*) during Smoltification', *Can. J. Zool.*, *61*, 1954.

McKeown, B.K. (1984) *Fish Migration*. Croom Helm, London; Timber Press, Portland, Oregon.

Mahnken, C., Prentice, E., Waknitz, W., Monan, G., Sims, C. and Williams, J. (1982) 'The Application of Recent Smoltification Research to Public Hatchery Releases: an Assessment of Size/time Requirements for Columbia River Hatchery Coho Salmon (*Oncorhynchus kisutch*)', *Aquaculture, 28*, 251.

Nagahama, Y., Clarke, C.W. and Hoar, W.S. (1977) 'Influence of Salinity on Ultrastructure of the Secretory Cells of the Adenohypophyseal Pars Distalis in Yearling Salmon (*Oncorhynchus kisutch*)', *Can. J. Zool.*, *55*, 183.

Nishiokka, R.S., Bern, H.A., Lai, K.V., Nagahama, Y. and Grau, E.G. (1982) 'Changes in the Endocrine Organs of Coho Salmon during Normal and Abnormal Smoltification — an Electron Microscope Study', *Aquaculture, 28*, 21.

Northcote, T.G. (1978) 'Migratory Strategies and Production in Freshwater Fishes' in S.D. Gerking (ed.), *Ecology of Freshwater Fish Production*, Blackwell, Oxford.

Polyakov, V.N. and Maximovich, A.A. (1980) 'A Morphometric Ultrastructural Study of Interrenal Tissue Cells at the Successive Stages of Spawning of the

Pink Salmon', *Tsitologiya, 22,* 907.

Specker, J.L. and Schrenk, C.B. (1982) 'Changes in Plasma Corticosteroids during Smoltification of Coho Salmon, *Oncorhynchus kisutch*', *Gen. Comp. Endocrinol., 46,* 53.

Thorpe, J.E. (ed.) (1980) *Salmon Ranching,* Academic Press, London.

Thorpe, J.E. and Morgan, R.I.G. (1978) 'Periodicity in Atlantic Salmon, *Salmo salar* L. Smolt Migration', *J. Fish Biol., 12,* 541.

Ueda, H., Hiroi, O., Hara, A, Yamauchi, K. and Nagahama, Y. (1984) 'Changes in Serum Concentrations of Steroid Hormones, Thyroxine and Vitellogenin during Spawning Migration of Chum Salmon, *Oncorhynchus keta*', *Gen. Comp. Endocrinol., 53,* 203.

Woodhead, A.D. (1959) 'Variations in the Activity of the Thyroid Gland of the Cod, *Gadus callarias* L. in Relation to Its Migrations in the Barents Sea', *J. Mar. Biol. Ass. UK, 38,* 407.

Chapter 9: Hormones and Aquaculture

Aida, K. (1978) 'Effect of LH-releasing Hormone on Gonadal Development in a Salmonid Fish, the Ayu', *Bull. Jap. Soc. Sci. Fish, 49,* 711.

Atz, J.W. and Pickford, G.E. (1964) 'The Pituitary Gland and its Relation to the Reproduction of Fishes in Nature and Captivity', *FAO Fish. Biol. tech. Pap.* (37), 61p.

Donaldson, E.M., (1982) 'Sex Control in Fish with Particular Reference to Salmonids', *Can. J. Fish. Aquat. Sci., 39,* 99.

Donaldson, E.M., Fagerlund, U.H.M., Higgs, D.A. and McBride, J.R. (1979) 'Hormonal Enhancement of Growth' in W.S. Hoar, D.J. Randall and J.R. Brett (eds.), *Fish Physiology,* Vol. 8, Academic Press, New York, p. 456.

Eckstein, B. and Spira, M. (1965) 'Effect of Sex Hormones on Gonadal Differentiation in a Cichlid, *Tilapia aurea*', *Biol. Bull., 129,* 482.

Fagerlund, U.H.M., Higgs, D.A., McBride, J.R., Plotnikoff, M.D., Dosanjh, B.S. and Markert, J.R. (1983) 'Implications of Varying Dietary Protein, Lipid and 17α-methyltestosterone Content on Growth and Utilization of Protein and Energy in Juvenile Coho Salmon (*Oncorhynchus kisutch*)', *Aquaculture, 30,* 109.

Fontaine, M. (1976) 'Hormones and the Control of Reproduction in Aquaculture', *J. Fish. Res. Board Can., 33,* 922.

Funk, J.D., Donaldson, E.M. and Dye, H.M. (1972) 'Induction of Precocious Sexual Development in Female Pink Salmon (*Oncorhynchus gorbuscha*)', *Can. J. Zool., 51,* 493.

Goetz, F.W., Donaldson, E.M., Hunter, G.A. and Dye, H.M. (1979) 'Effect of Oestradiol-17β and 17α-methyltestosterone on Gonadal Differentiation in the Coho Salmon, *Oncorhynchus kisutch. Aquaculture, 17,* 267.

Guerrero, R.D. (1975) 'Use of Androgens for the Production of All-male *Tilapia aurea*', *Trans. Am. Fish. Soc., 2,* 342.

Habibi, H.R., Ince, B.W. and Matty, A.J. (1983) 'Effects of 17α-methyltestosterone and 17β-oestradiol on Intestinal Transport and Absorption of ¹⁴C-leucine *in vitro* in Rainbow Trout (*Salmo gairdneri*), *J. Comp. Physiol., 151,* 247.

Higgs, D.A., Fagerlund, U.H.M., Eales, J.G. and McBride, J.R. (1982) 'Application of Thyroid and Steroid Hormones as Anabolic Agents in Fish Culture', *Comp. Biochem. Physiol., 73B,* 143.

Higgs, D.A., Fagerlund, U.H.M., McBride, J.R. and Eales, J.G. (1979) 'Influence

258   Bibliography

of Orally Administered 1-thyroxine or 3, 5, 3'-triiodo-1-thyronine on Growth, Food Consumption, and Food Conversion of Under-yearling Coho Salmon (*Oncorhynchus kisutch*)', *Can. J. Zool.*, 57, 1974.

Hirose, K., Machida, Y. and Donaldson, E.M. (1979) 'Induced Ovulation of Japanese Flounder with Human Chorionic Gonadotropin and Salmon Gonadotropin with Special Reference to Changes in Quality of Eggs Retained in the Ovarian Cavity after Ovulation', *Bull. Jap. Soc. Sci. Fish.*, 45, 31.

Hunt, S.M.V., Simpson, T.H. and Wright, R.S. (1982) 'Seasonal Changes in the Levels of 11-oxotestosterone and Testosterone in the Serum of Male Salmon, *Salmo salar L.*, and Their Relationship to Growth and Maturation Cycle', *J. Fish. Biol.*, 20, 105.

Hunter, G.A., Donaldson, E.M. and Dye, H.M. (1981) 'Induced Ovulation in Coho Salmon: 1. Further Studies on the Use of Salmon Pituitary Preparations', *Aquaculture*, 26, 117.

Jalabert, B., Breton, B., Brzuka, E., Fostier, A. and Wieniawski, J. (1977) 'A New Tool for Inducing Spawning: the Use of 17α-hydroxy-20β-dihydroprogesterone to Spawn Carp at Low Temperature', *Aquaculture*, 10, 353.

Jensen, G.L. and Shelton, W.L. (1979) 'Effects of Estrogens on *Tilapia aurea*: Implications for Production of Monosex Genetic Male Tilapia. *Aquaculture*, 16, 233.

Jensen, G.L., Shelton, W.L., Yang, S. and Wilken, L.O. (1983) 'Sex Reversal of Gynogenetic Grass Carp by Implantation of Methyltestosterone', *Trans. Am. Fish. Soc.*, 112, 79.

Johnstone, R., Simpson, T.H. and Walker, A.F. (1979) 'Sex Reversal in Salmonid Culture. Part 3. The Production and Performance of All-female Populations of Brook Trout', *Aquaculture*, 18, 241.

Johnstone, R., Simpson, T.H. and Youngson, A.F. (1978) 'Sex Reversal in Salmonid Culture', *Aquaculture*, 13, 115.

Jungwirth, M. (1979) 'Ovulation Inducement in Prespawning Adult Danube Salmon (*Hucho hucho L.*) by Injection of Acetone Dried Carp Pituitary (CP)', *Aquaculture*, 17, 129.

Laird, L.M., Wilson, A.R. and Holliday, F.G.T. (1980) 'Field Trials of a Method of Induction of Autoimmune Gonad Rejection in Atlantic Salmon (*Salmo salar L.*)', *Reprod. Nutr. Develop.*, 20, 1781.

Lam, T.J. (1982) 'Applications of Endocrinology to Fish Culture', *Can. J. Fish. Aquat. Sci.*, 39, 111.

Lone, K.P. and Ince, B.W. (1983) 'Cellular Growth Responses of Rainbow Trout (*Salmo gairdneri*) Fed Different Levels of Dietary Protein and an Anabolic Steroid Ethylestrenol', *Gen. Comp. Endocrinol.*, 49, 32.

Lone, K.P. and Matty, A.J. (1980) 'The Effect of Feeding Methyltestosterone on the Growth and Body Composition of Common Carp (*Cyprinus carpio L.*)', *Gen. Comp. Endocrinol.*, 40, 409.

Lone, K.P. and Matty, A.J. (1981) 'The Effect of Feeding Androgenic Hormones on the Proteolytic Activity of the Alimentary Canal of Carp, *Cyprinus carpio L.*', *J. Fish. Biol.*, 18, 353.

Matty, A.J. and Cheema, I.R. (1978) 'The Effect of Some Steroid Hormones on the Growth and Protein Metabolism of Rainbow Trout', *Aquaculture*, 14, 163.

McBride, J.R. and Fagerlund, U.H.M. (1973) 'The Use of 17α-methyltestosterone for Promoting Weight Increases in Juvenile Pacific Salmon', *J. Fish. Res. Board Can.*, 30, 1099.

Murat, J.C., Plisetskaya, E.M. and Woo, N.Y.S. (1981) 'Endocrine Control of Nutrition in Cyclostomes and Fish', *Comp. Biochem. Physiol.*, 68A, 149.

Payne, A.I. (1979) 'Physiological and Ecological Factors in the Development of Fish Culture', *Symp. Zool. Soc. Lond.*, 44, 383.

Richter, C.J.J. and van den Hurk, R. (1982) 'Effects of 11-desoxycorticosterone-acetate and Carp Pituitary Suspension on Follicle Maturation in the Ovaries of the African Catfish, *Clarias lazera (C. & V.)* ', *Aquaculture, 29*, 53.

Rothbard, S. and Pruginin, Y. (1975) 'Induced Spawning and Artificial Incubation of *Tilapia*', *Aquaculture, 5*, 315.

Saunders, R.L., Henderson, E.B. and Glebe, B.D. (1982) 'Precocious Sexual Maturation and Smoltification in Male Atlantic Salmon (*Salmo salar*)', *Aquaculture, 28*, 211.

Schreck, C.B. (1982) 'Stress and Rearing of Salmonids', *Aquaculture, 28*, 241.

Schreck, C.B. and Fowler, L.G. (1981/1982) 'Growth and Reproductive Development in Fall Chinook Salmon: Effects of Sex Hormones and Their Antagonists', *Aquaculture, 26*, 253.

Simpson, T.H. (1975/1976) 'Endocrine Aspects of Salmonid Culture', *Proc. Roy. Soc. Edinburgh* (B), *75*, 241.

Sower, S.A. and Schreck, C.B. (1982) '*In vitro* Induction of Final Maturation of Oocytes from Coho Salmon', *Trans. Am. Fish. Soc., 111*, 399.

Sower, S.A., Schreck, C.B. and Donaldson, E.M. (1982) 'Hormone-induced Ovulation of Coho Salmon (*Oncorhynchus kisutch*) Held in Seawater and Fresh Water', *Can. J. Fish. Aquat. Sci., 39*, 627.

Van Der Kraak, G., Lin, H., Donaldson, E.M., Dye, H.M. and Hunter, G. (1983) 'Effects of LH-RH and des-Gly. [D-Ala]LH-RH-ethylamide on Plasma Gonadotropin Levels and Oocyte Maturation in Adult Female Coho Salmon (*Oncorhynchus kisutch*)', *Gen. Comp. Endocrinol., 49*, 470.

Wright, R.S. and Hunt, S.M.V. (1982) 'A Radioimmunoassay for 17α, 20β-dihydroxy-4-pregnen-3-one: its Use in Measuring Changes in Serum Levels at Ovulation in Atlantic Salmon (*Salmo salar*), Coho Salmon (*Oncorhynchus kisutch*), and Rainbow Trout (*Salmo gairdneri*)', *Gen. Comp. Endocrinol., 47*, 475.

Yamamoto, K., Morioka, T., Hiroi, O. and Omori, M. (1974) 'Artificial Maturation of Female Japanese Eels by the Injection of Salmonid Pituitary', *Bull. Jap. Soc. Sci. Fish., 40*, 1.

GENERAL INDEX

FISH SPECIES INDEX